MY ENABLED WARRIOR TRACKER

WE PUSH THE LIMITS

WE MAKE CHANGE HAPPEN

WE ARE MENTALLY STRONG

WE CAN DO ANYTHING

We are ENabled warriors

Join the Tribe on Facebook search ENabled Warriors!

Written and designed by Jessie Ace

Hey Warrior!

This book is designed to help you feel empowered. It is not a quick fix, it will take dedication and practice to make sure you fill it in every day, it should only take you around 5 minutes and you can take more time or less time depending on your day and energy level.

I know first hand how hard it is to live with a chronic illness, remembering all those countless appointments, when symptoms started and the date of your last relapse can be tough. This book will make appointments far easier.

If you need some help to stay positive this book is for you.

The book is split into daily, weekly and monthly sheets to help you track your symptoms and to find triggers.

Keep track of symptoms on your daily sheets (noting the severity level) and add these to your 1 month graph and your 3 month graph so you can track of everything that's happened and you can take accurate info to your medical team.

If it seems overwhelming, start small. Fill in one section or one page per day. You are in control of when you start the book.

Get ready to be your medical teams star patient!

I was diagnosed at 22 with Multiple Sclerosis

Tips and Tricks

Look through the whole book before starting So you fill everything in. If it feels overwhelming, start with just one section of one page and build from there.

Use post it notes to mark your pages so you can always find everything

Filling in this tracker is part of your daily 'me time'. Have fun with it and enjoy!

Let's be friends

FB Group: /groups/ENabledwarriors
FB page: DISabledtoENabled
Instagram: DISabledtoENabled

Ps. You can do anything

HOW TO USE THIS BOOK

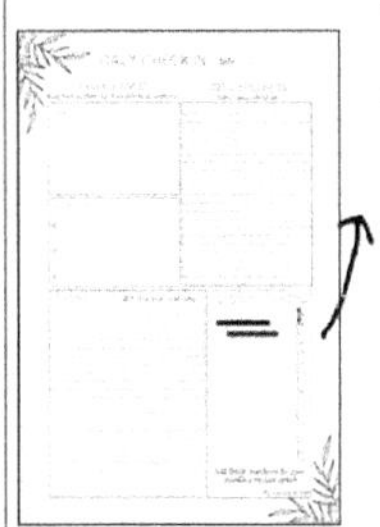

Fill in your symptoms on the daily sheet. Give it a score out of 10 for the day (10 = worst) and add this number to your 1 month graph using different coloured lines for each symptom.. At the end of the week add up all your numbers and divide by 7 (7 days in a week). This is your weekly average number.

Add your weekly average number on your 3 month review graph. Again, use a different coloured line for each symptom.

Tip: If you have numbers like 10.83 round your numbers up or down to the closest whole number. E.g. 10.83 would be 11.

Adding your info onto the graph helps you see what is improving, and helps your health care team determine what help you need (without you having to remember a thing, Boom!) There's also a sheet for your medical history quick notes so if you're ever caught off guard in an appointment, no worries everything is on hand.

Add your daily symptom number to your 1 month review page at the start of each month. From there you can see an average of how your symptoms have behaved over the month.

Use the other tracker sheets in this book like the food diary to find a pattern for why your symptoms fluctuated.Remember to make a note of this for your next appointment.

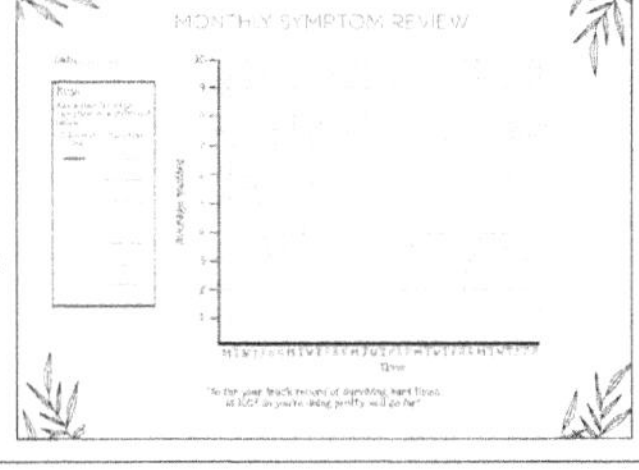

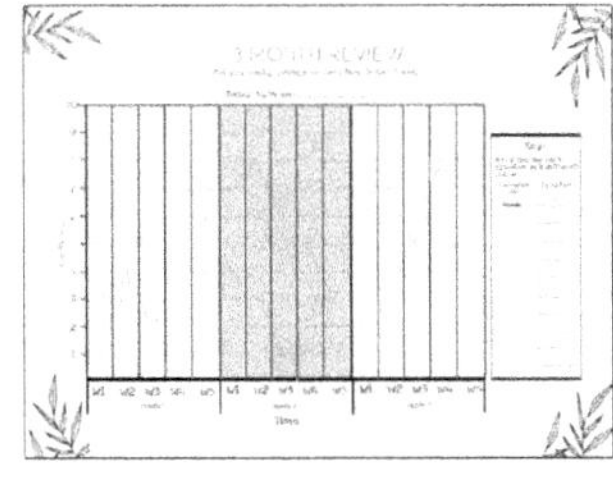

Add your weekly average numbers from the end of week review page to your 3 month graph at the start of this book.

This helps your medical professionals get a quick overview of how you've been doing and you can write notes when you think of things to ask them.

3 MONTH REVIEW

Plot your weekly average numbers here to spot trends

Dates from and to: ____________________

Severity level

10
9
8
7
6
5
4
3
2
1

W1	W2	W3	W4	W5	W1	W2	W3	W4	W5	W1	W2	W3	W4	W5
Month 1					Month 2					Month 3				

Week/Month

Fatigue
Pain

Key (use a different colour line for each symptom)

Line	Symptom

Key points to discuss

USEFUL DETAILS

This book belongs to: ____________________

Medical conditions: ____________________

____

____

	Address	Phone number	Email Address

Ps You can do anything

MEDICAL RECORD QUICK NOTES

My Blood Type: ____________________ My allergies: ____________________

____

Date	Diagnosed with	Doctor/hospital	Treatment

SURGICAL PROCEDURES / TESTS

Date	Diagnosed with	Doctor/hospital	Treatment

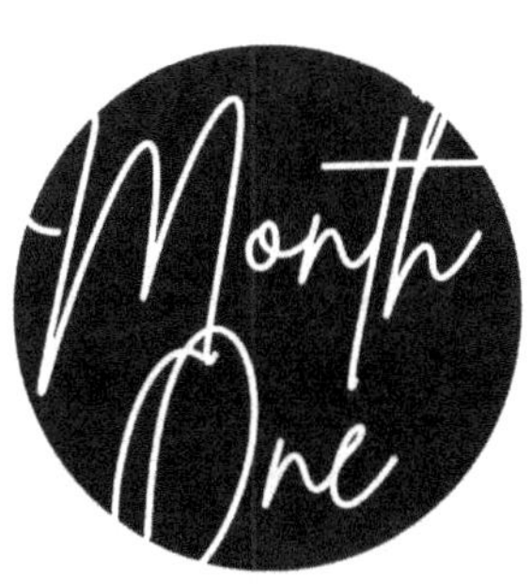

Let's do this!

"Success is 80% psychology" - Tony Robbins

Remember to fill in those daily sheets!

What word are you choosing for this month to focus your energy?

My word for this month is...

CALENDAR

Month: ....

M	T	W	T	F	S	S

I need to remember:

APPOINTMENT TRACKER

Appointment with:

On:

At:

My treat after will be:

Remember

- [ ]
- [ ]
- [ ]
- [ ]
- [ ]

Remember to ask/tell them about:

They Said:

APPOINTMENT TRACKER

Appointment with:

On:

At:

My treat after will be:

Remember

- [ ]
- [ ]
- [ ]
- [ ]
- [ ]

Remember to ask/tell them about:

They said:

APPOINTMENT TRACKER

Appointment with:

On:

At:

My treat after will be:

Remember

- [ ]
- [ ]
- [ ]
- [ ]
- [ ]

Remember to ask/tell them about:

They said:

APPOINTMENT TRACKER

Appointment with:

On:

At:

My treat after will be:

Remember

- [ ]
- [ ]
- [ ]
- [ ]
- [ ]

Remember to ask/tell them about:

They said:

1 MONTH REVIEW

Take the numbers from your daily sheets and plot them on this graph to help your medical professional get a quick glance of your health

Dates from and to: ______________________

Average number

10
9
8
7
6
5
4
3
2
1

M T W T F S S M T W T F S S M T W T F S S M T W T F S S M T W T F S S

Day

Make a note of the date under the day

Key (use a different colour line for each symptom)

Line	Symptom

Key points to discuss

You have a 100% track record for survivng the bad times, that's pretty good going!

EXERCISE TRACKER

Track your exercise progress in each of the boxes, write the activity that you did.
Make sure to write in your goal at the bottom!

Start

Finish

My goal is:

MENSTRUAL TRACKER

Month..

Key = ◩ = Normal Flow ■ = Heavy Flow ⊡ = Spotting

M	T	W	T	F	S	S

Add the calendar dates into the boxes of the month so you can see any patterns between symptoms

GOAL TRACKER

Have goals you want to complete this month? This is for you.
Add your goals to the bottom of the page so you can work backwards to work out what you need to do to reach that goal

Start

Finish

My goals are:

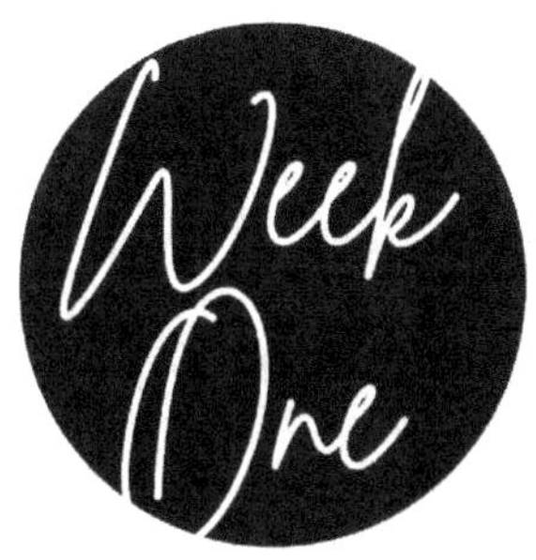

Let's get stuck in to week 1 warrior!

Check through the whole weeks sheets before starting so you don't miss anything

Quote for the week:

You can't worry about something that you have no control over.

PILL / SUPPLEMENT TRACKER

key:

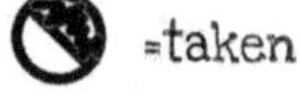 =taken

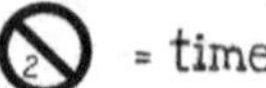 = time

Use different colours for different medications

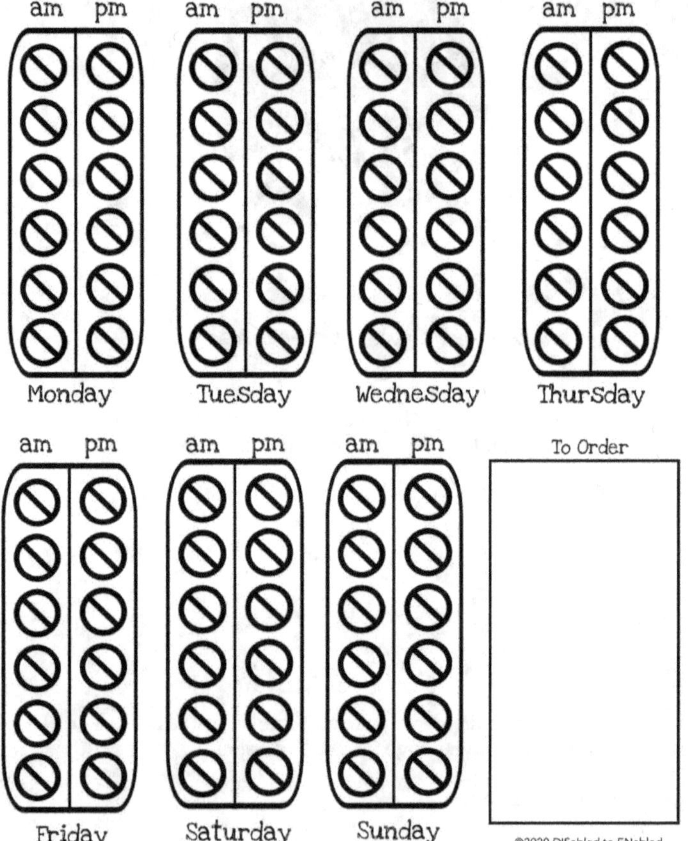

To Order

"I can handle anything"

TREATMENT DIARY

Treatment ______________________ Start date: ___________

Date	Dose	pre/post meds taken	Reactions/ side effects	My treat will be

"What doesn't challenge us, doesn't change us"
You can do this.

TREATMENT DIARY

Treatment ____________________ Start date: __________

Date	Dose	pre/post meds taken	Reactions/ side effects	My treat will be

"What doesn't challenge us, doesn't change us"
You can do this.

FOOD DIARY

	Monday	Tuesday	Wednesday	Thursday	Friday	Saturday	Sunday
Breakfast							
Snacks							
Lunch							
Snacks							
Dinner							
Snacks							

HYDRATION TRACKER

Grab a big bottle of water and add the amount of water you've drank in a day.

M	T	W	T	F	S	S

DAILY CHECK IN

Date:...

DAILY 'I AM'S'

Keep them positive! E.g. 'I am able to do anything'

I AM...

I AM...

I AM...

I AM...

I AM...

TODAY'S PRIORITIES:

★

★

★

GRATEFULNESS

Today I am grateful for...

JOURNAL SPACE: What is on your mind today?

SYMPTOMS I FEEL TODAY

Rate each symptom in severity from 1-10. 1 being low and 10 is high

Add these numbers to your monthly review graph

P.S. You can do this!

DAILY CHECK IN

Date:..

DAILY 'I AM'S'

Keep them positive! E.g. 'I am able to do anything'

I AM...

I AM...

I AM...

I AM...

I AM...

GRATEFULNESS

Today I am grateful for...

TODAY'S PRIORITIES:

★

★

★

JOURNAL SPACE: What is on your mind today?

SYMPTOMS I FEEL TODAY

Rate each symptom in severity from 1-10 1 being low and 10 is high

Add these numbers to your monthly review graph

P.S. You can do this!

DAILY CHECK IN

Date:..

DAILY 'I AM'S'

Keep them positive! E.g. 'I am able to do anything'

I AM...

I AM...

I AM...

I AM...

I AM...

GRATEFULNESS

Today I am grateful for...

TODAY'S PRIORITIES:

★

★

★

JOURNAL SPACE: What is on your mind today?

SYMPTOMS I FEEL TODAY

Rate each symptom in severity from 1-10. 1 being low and 10 is high

Add these numbers to your monthly review graph

P.S. You can do this!

DAILY CHECK IN

Date:..

DAILY 'I AM'S'

Keep them positive! E.g. 'I am able to do anything'

I AM...

I AM...

I AM...

I AM...

I AM...

TODAY'S PRIORITIES:

★

★

★

GRATEFULNESS

Today I am grateful for...

JOURNAL SPACE: What is on your mind today?

SYMPTOMS I FEEL TODAY

Rate each symptom in severity from 1-10. 1 being low and 10 is high

Add these numbers to your monthly review graph

P.S. You can do this!

DAILY CHECK IN

Date:..

DAILY 'I AM'S'

Keep them positive! E.g. 'I am able to do anything'

I AM...

I AM...

I AM...

I AM...

I AM...

GRATEFULNESS

Today I am grateful for...

TODAY'S PRIORITIES:

★

★

★

JOURNAL SPACE: What is on your mind today?

SYMPTOMS I FEEL TODAY

Rate each symptom in severity from 1-10. 1 being low and 10 is high

Add these numbers to your monthly review graph

P.S. You can do this!

DAILY CHECK IN

Date:..

DAILY 'I AM'S'

Keep them positive! E.g. 'I am able to do anything'

I AM...

I AM...

I AM...

I AM...

I AM...

GRATEFULNESS

Today I am grateful for...

TODAY'S PRIORITIES:

★

★

★

JOURNAL SPACE: What is on your mind today?

SYMPTOMS I FEEL TODAY

Rate each symptom in severity from 1-10 1 being low and 10 is high

Add these numbers to your monthly review graph

P.S. You can do this!

DAILY CHECK IN   Date:..

DAILY 'I AM'S'
Keep them positive! E.g. 'I am able to do anything'

I AM...

I AM...

I AM...

I AM...

I AM...

GRATEFULNESS
Today I am grateful for...

TODAY'S PRIORITIES:

★

★

★

JOURNAL SPACE: What is on your mind today?

SYMPTOMS I FEEL TODAY
Rate each symptom in severity from 1-10. 1 being low and 10 is high

Add these numbers to your monthly review graph

P.S. You can do this!

END OF WEEK REVIEW

Symptom.......................

M	T	W	T	F	S	S	Weekly Average*

Symptom.......................

M	T	W	T	F	S	S	Weekly Average*

Symptom.......................

M	T	W	T	F	S	S	Weekly Average*

Symptom.......................

M	T	W	T	F	S	S	Weekly Average*

Symptom.......................

M	T	W	T	F	S	S	Weekly Average*

Remember to add Monday to Sunday rating onto your graph on the monthly review page

And add the weekly average to your 3 month graph at the start of this book

Meds I took this week:

Achievements

Challenges faced

Things to order (medication/equipment/etc)

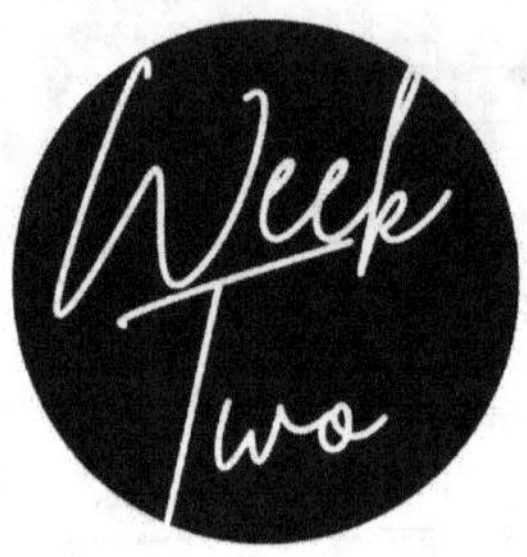

These are your pages to be filled in after a week.

You'll find a medication sheet, timetable, food diary, mood tracker, sleep tracker and dream diary.

These sheets combined keep you organised and in control.

Use these sheets for creating patterns between different things.

Tip: Fill in daily if you think you may not remember, otherwise fill this in on a Sunday eve to be ready for the next week.

PILL / SUPPLEMENT TRACKER

key:

 =taken  = time Use different colours for different medications

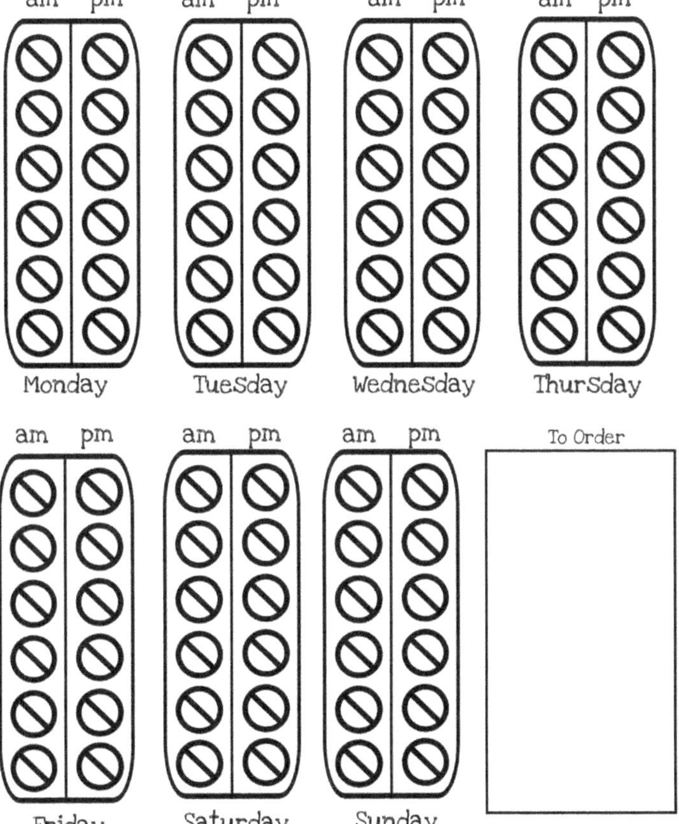

"I can handle anything"

TREATMENT DIARY

Treatment ____________________ Start date: __________

Date	Dose	pre/post meds taken	Reactions/ side effects	My treat will be

"What doesn't challenge us, doesn't change us"
You can do this.

TREATMENT DIARY

Treatment ______________________ Start date: ___________

Date	Dose	pre/post meds taken	Reactions/ side effects	My treat will be

"What doesn't challenge us, doesn't change us"
You can do this.

FOOD DIARY

	Monday	Tuesday	Wednesday	Thursday	Friday	Saturday	Sunday
Breakfast							
Snacks							
Lunch							
Snacks							
Dinner							
Snacks							

HYDRATION TRACKER

Grab a big bottle of water and add the amount of water you've drank in a day.

M	T	W	T	F	S	S

DAILY CHECK IN

Date:..

DAILY 'I AM'S'

Keep them positive! E.g. 'I am able to do anything'

I AM...

I AM...

I AM...

I AM...

I AM...

GRATEFULNESS

Today I am grateful for...

TODAY'S PRIORITIES:

★

★

★

JOURNAL SPACE: What is on your mind today?

SYMPTOMS I FEEL TODAY

Rate each symptom in severity from 1-10. 1 being low and 10 is high

Add these numbers to your monthly review graph

P.S. You can do this!

DAILY CHECK IN

Date:..

DAILY 'I AM'S'

Keep them positive! E.g. 'I am able to do anything'

I AM...

I AM...

I AM...

I AM...

I AM...

GRATEFULNESS

Today I am grateful for...

TODAY'S PRIORITIES:

★

★

★

JOURNAL SPACE: What is on your mind today?

SYMPTOMS I FEEL TODAY

Rate each symptom in severity from 1-10. 1 being low and 10 is high

Add these numbers to your monthly review graph

P.S. You can do this!

DAILY CHECK IN

Date:..

DAILY 'I AM'S'

Keep them positive! E.g. 'I am able to do anything'

I AM...

I AM...

I AM...

I AM...

I AM...

TODAY'S PRIORITIES:

★

★

★

GRATEFULNESS

Today I am grateful for...

JOURNAL SPACE: What is on your mind today?

SYMPTOMS I FEEL TODAY

Rate each symptom in severity from 1-10. 1 being low and 10 is high

Add these numbers to your monthly review graph

P.S. You can do this!

DAILY CHECK IN Date:...

DAILY 'I AM'S'

Keep them positive! E.g. 'I am able to do anything'

I AM...

I AM...

I AM...

I AM...

I AM...

TODAY'S PRIORITIES:

★

★

★

GRATEFULNESS

Today I am grateful for...

JOURNAL SPACE: What is on your mind today?

SYMPTOMS I FEEL TODAY

Rate each symptom in severity from 1-10. 1 being low and 10 is high

Add these numbers to your monthly review graph

P.S. You can do this!

DAILY CHECK IN

Date:..

DAILY 'I AM'S'

Keep them positive! E.g. 'I am able to do anything'

I AM...

I AM...

I AM...

I AM...

I AM...

GRATEFULNESS

Today I am grateful for...

TODAY'S PRIORITIES:

★

★

★

JOURNAL SPACE: What is on your mind today?

SYMPTOMS I FEEL TODAY

Rate each symptom in severity from 1-10. 1 being low and 10 is high

Add these numbers to your monthly review graph

P.S. You can do this!

DAILY CHECK IN

Date:..

DAILY 'I AM'S'

Keep them positive! E.g. 'I am able to do anything'

I AM...

I AM...

I AM...

I AM...

I AM...

GRATEFULNESS

Today I am grateful for...

TODAY'S PRIORITIES:

★

★

★

JOURNAL SPACE: What is on your mind today?

SYMPTOMS I FEEL TODAY

Rate each symptom in severity from 1-10. 1 being low and 10 is high

Add these numbers to your monthly review graph

P.S. You can do this!

DAILY CHECK IN

Date:..

DAILY 'I AM'S'

Keep them positive! E.g. 'I am able to do anything'

I AM...

I AM...

I AM...

I AM...

I AM...

GRATEFULNESS

Today I am grateful for...

TODAY'S PRIORITIES:

★

★

★

JOURNAL SPACE: What is on your mind today?

SYMPTOMS I FEEL TODAY

Rate each symptom in severity from 1-10 1 being low and 10 is high

Add these numbers to your monthly review graph

P.S. You can do this!

END OF WEEK REVIEW

Symptom.........................

M	T	W	T	F	S	S	Weekly Average*

Symptom.........................

M	T	W	T	F	S	S	Weekly Average*

Symptom.........................

M	T	W	T	F	S	S	Weekly Average*

Symptom.........................

M	T	W	T	F	S	S	Weekly Average*

Symptom.........................

M	T	W	T	F	S	S	Weekly Average*

Remember to add Monday to Sunday rating onto your graph on the monthly review page

And add the weekly average to your 3 month graph at the start of this book.

Meds I took this week:

Achievements

Challenges faced

Things to order (medication/equipment/etc)

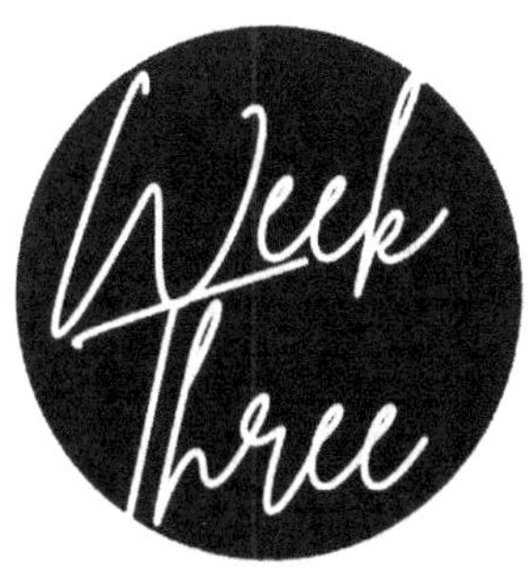

Let's get stuck in to week 3 warrior!

Check through the whole weeks sheets before starting so you don't miss anything

Quote for the week:

How would the person I want to be, do the things that I want to do now?

PILL / SUPPLEMENT TRACKER

key:

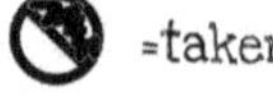

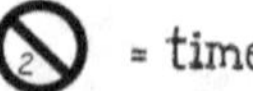

Use different colours for different medications

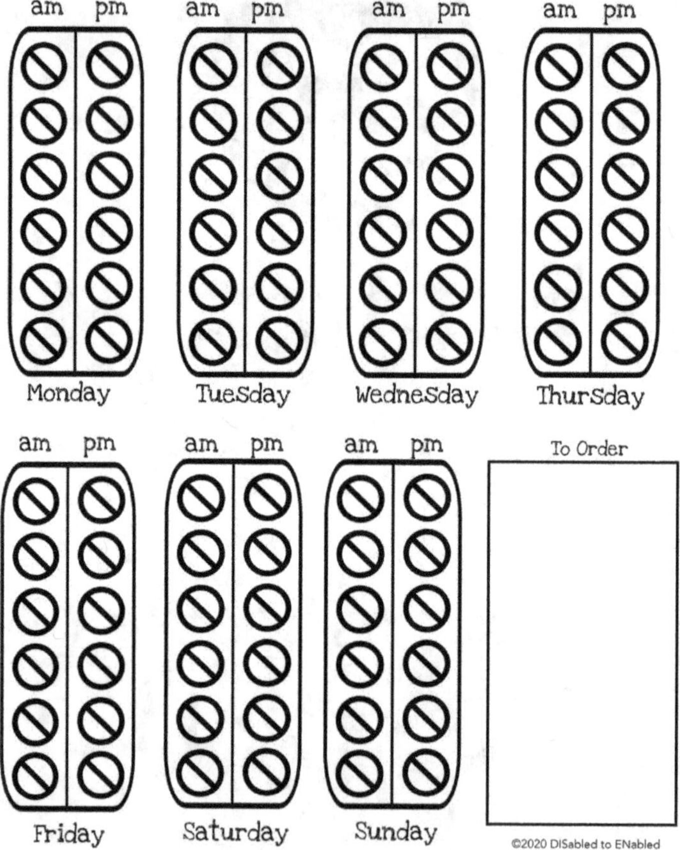

"I can handle anything"

TREATMENT DIARY

Treatment ____________________ Start date: __________

Date	Dose	pre/post meds taken	Reactions/ Side effects	My treat will be

"What doesn't challenge us, doesn't change us"
You can do this.

TREATMENT DIARY

Treatment ____________________ Start date: __________

Date	Dose	pre/post meds taken	Reactions/ side effects	My treat will be

"What doesn't challenge us, doesn't change us"
You can do this.

FOOD DIARY

	Monday	Tuesday	Wednesday	Thursday	Friday	Saturday	Sunday
Breakfast							
Snacks							
Lunch							
Snacks							
Dinner							
Snacks							

HYDRATION TRACKER

Grab a big bottle of water and add the amount of water you've drank in a day.

M	T	W	T	F	S	S

DAILY CHECK IN

Date:..

DAILY 'I AM'S'

Keep them positive! E.g. 'I am able to do anything'

I AM...

I AM...

I AM...

I AM...

I AM...

GRATEFULNESS

Today I am grateful for...

TODAY'S PRIORITIES:

★

★

★

JOURNAL SPACE: What is on your mind today?

SYMPTOMS I FEEL TODAY

Rate each symptom in severity from 1-10. 1 being low and 10 is high

Add these numbers to your monthly review graph

P.S. You can do this!

DAILY CHECK IN

Date:..

DAILY 'I AM'S'

Keep them positive! E.g. 'I am able to do anything'

I AM...

I AM...

I AM...

I AM...

I AM...

GRATEFULNESS

Today I am grateful for...

TODAY'S PRIORITIES:

★

★

★

JOURNAL SPACE: What is on your mind today?

SYMPTOMS I FEEL TODAY

Rate each symptom in severity from 1-10. 1 being low and 10 is high

Add these numbers to your monthly review graph

P.S. You can do this!

DAILY CHECK IN

Date:...

DAILY 'I AM'S'

Keep them positive! E.g. 'I am able to do anything'

I AM...

I AM...

I AM...

I AM...

I AM...

GRATEFULNESS

Today I am grateful for...

TODAY'S PRIORITIES:

★

★

★

JOURNAL SPACE: What is on your mind today?

SYMPTOMS I FEEL TODAY

Rate each symptom in severity from 1-10. 1 being low and 10 is high

Add these numbers to your monthly review graph

P.S. You can do this!

DAILY CHECK IN

Date:..

DAILY 'I AM'S'

Keep them positive! E.g. 'I am able to do anything'

I AM...

I AM...

I AM...

I AM...

I AM...

GRATEFULNESS

Today I am grateful for...

TODAY'S PRIORITIES:

★

★

★

JOURNAL SPACE: What is on your mind today?

SYMPTOMS I FEEL TODAY

Rate each symptom in severity from 1-10. 1 being low and 10 is high

Add these numbers to your monthly review graph

P.S. You can do this!

DAILY CHECK IN

Date:..

DAILY 'I AM'S'

Keep them positive! E.g. 'I am able to do anything'

I AM...

I AM...

I AM...

I AM...

I AM...

GRATEFULNESS

Today I am grateful for...

TODAY'S PRIORITIES:

★

★

★

JOURNAL SPACE: What is on your mind today?

SYMPTOMS I FEEL TODAY

Rate each Symptom in Severity from 1-10. 1 being low and 10 is high

Add these numbers to your monthly review graph

P.S. You can do this!

DAILY CHECK IN

Date:...

DAILY 'I AM'S'

Keep them positive! E.g. 'I am able to do anything'

I AM...

I AM...

I AM...

I AM...

I AM...

TODAY'S PRIORITIES:

★

★

★

GRATEFULNESS

Today I am grateful for...

JOURNAL SPACE: What is on your mind today?

SYMPTOMS I FEEL TODAY

Rate each symptom in severity from 1-10 1 being low and 10 is high

Add these numbers to your monthly review graph

P.S. You can do this!

DAILY CHECK IN

Date:..

DAILY 'I AM'S'

Keep them positive! E.g. 'I am able to do anything'

I AM...

I AM...

I AM...

I AM...

I AM...

GRATEFULNESS

Today I am grateful for...

TODAY'S PRIORITIES:

★

★

★

JOURNAL SPACE: What is on your mind today?

SYMPTOMS I FEEL TODAY

Rate each symptom in severity from 1-10. 1 being low and 10 is high

Add these numbers to your monthly review graph

P.S. You can do this!

END OF WEEK REVIEW

Symptom.........................

M T W T F S S

Weekly Average*

Symptom.........................

M T W T F S S

Weekly Average*

Symptom.........................

M T W T F S S

Weekly Average*

Symptom.........................

M T W T F S S

Weekly Average*

Symptom.........................

M T W T F S S

Weekly Average*

Remember to add Monday to Sunday rating onto your graph on the monthly review page

And add the weekly average to your 3 month graph at the start of this book.

Meds I took this week:

Achievements

Challenges faced

Things to order (medication/equipment/etc)

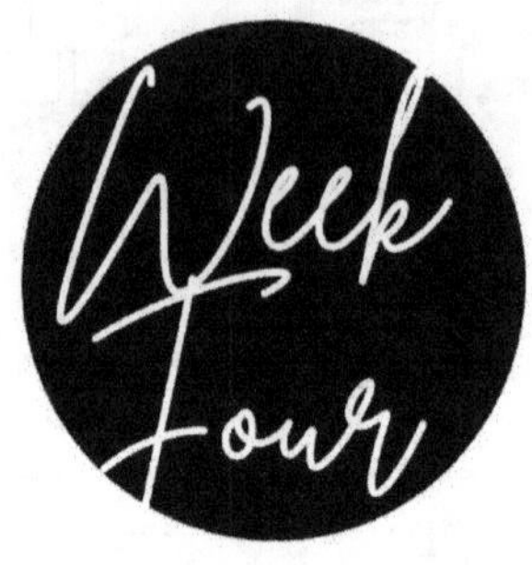

Let's get stuck in to week 4 warrior!

Check through the whole weeks sheets before starting so you don't miss anything

Quote for the week:

As long as you breathe you got a shot at your dream.

PILL / SUPPLEMENT TRACKER

key:

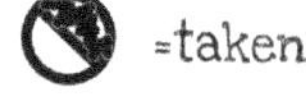
=taken

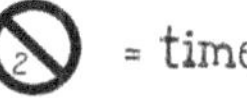
= time

Use different colours for different medications

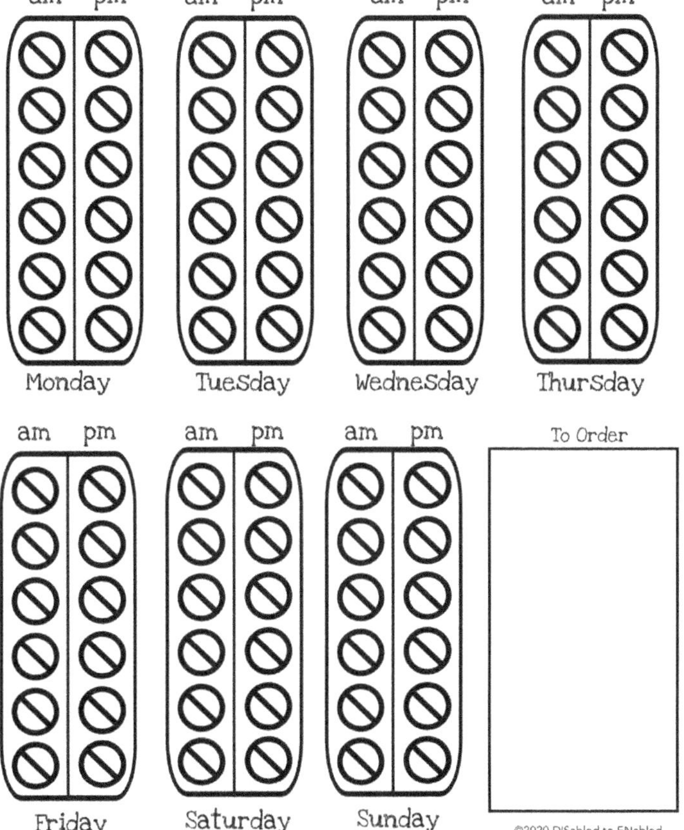

To Order

"I can handle anything"

TREATMENT DIARY

Treatment ______________________ Start date: ___________

Date	Dose	pre/post meds taken	Reactions/ Side effects	My treat will be

"What doesn't challenge us, doesn't change us"
You can do this.

TREATMENT DIARY

Treatment ______________________ Start date: ___________

Date	Dose	pre/post meds taken	Reactions/ side effects	My treat will be

"What doesn't challenge us, doesn't change us"
You can do this.

FOOD DIARY

	Monday	Tuesday	Wednesday	Thursday	Friday	Saturday	Sunday
Breakfast							
Snacks							
Lunch							
Snacks							
Dinner							
Snacks							

HYDRATION TRACKER

Grab a big bottle of water and add the amount of water you've drank in a day.

M	T	W	T	F	S	S

DAILY CHECK IN

Date:..

DAILY 'I AM'S'

Keep them positive! E.g. 'I am able to do anything'

I AM...

I AM...

I AM...

I AM...

I AM...

GRATEFULNESS

Today I am grateful for...

TODAY'S PRIORITIES:

★

★

★

JOURNAL SPACE: What is on your mind today?

SYMPTOMS I FEEL TODAY

Rate each symptom in severity from 1-10. 1 being low and 10 is high

Add these numbers to your monthly review graph

P.S. You can do this!

DAILY CHECK IN

Date:...

DAILY 'I AM'S'

Keep them positive! E.g. 'I am able to do anything'

I AM...

I AM...

I AM...

I AM...

I AM...

GRATEFULNESS

Today I am grateful for...

TODAY'S PRIORITIES:

★

★

★

JOURNAL SPACE: What is on your mind today?

SYMPTOMS I FEEL TODAY

Rate each symptom in severity from 1-10. 1 being low and 10 is high

Add these numbers to your monthly review graph

P.S. You can do this!

DAILY CHECK IN

Date:..

DAILY 'I AM'S'

Keep them positive! E.g. 'I am able to do anything'

I AM...

I AM...

I AM...

I AM...

I AM...

GRATEFULNESS

Today I am grateful for...

TODAY'S PRIORITIES:

★

★

★

JOURNAL SPACE: What is on your mind today?

SYMPTOMS I FEEL TODAY

Rate each symptom in severity from 1-10. 1 being low and 10 is high

Add these numbers to your monthly review graph

P.S. You can do this!

DAILY CHECK IN

Date:...

DAILY 'I AM'S'

Keep them positive! E.g. 'I am able to do anything'

I AM...

I AM...

I AM...

I AM...

I AM...

GRATEFULNESS

Today I am grateful for...

TODAY'S PRIORITIES:

★

★

★

JOURNAL SPACE: What is on your mind today?

SYMPTOMS I FEEL TODAY

Rate each symptom in severity from 1-10. 1 being low and 10 is high

Add these numbers to your monthly review graph

P.S. You can do this!

DAILY CHECK IN

Date:...

DAILY 'I AM'S'

Keep them positive! E.g. 'I am able to do anything'

I AM...

I AM...

I AM...

I AM...

I AM...

GRATEFULNESS

Today I am grateful for...

TODAY'S PRIORITIES:

★

★

★

JOURNAL SPACE: What is on your mind today?

SYMPTOMS I FEEL TODAY

Rate each symptom in severity from 1-10 1 being low and 10 is high

Add these numbers to your monthly review graph

P.S. You can do this!

DAILY CHECK IN

Date:..

DAILY 'I AM'S'

Keep them positive! E.g. 'I am able to do anything'

I AM...

I AM...

I AM...

I AM...

I AM...

TODAY'S PRIORITIES:

★

★

★

GRATEFULNESS

Today I am grateful for...

JOURNAL SPACE: What is on your mind today?

SYMPTOMS I FEEL TODAY

Rate each symptom in severity from 1-10. 1 being low and 10 is high

Add these numbers to your monthly review graph

P.S. You can do this!

DAILY CHECK IN

Date:...

DAILY 'I AM'S'

Keep them positive! E.g. 'I am able to do anything'

I AM...

I AM...

I AM...

I AM...

I AM...

GRATEFULNESS

Today I am grateful for...

TODAY'S PRIORITIES:

★

★

★

JOURNAL SPACE: What is on your mind today?

SYMPTOMS I FEEL TODAY

Rate each symptom in severity from 1-10. 1 being low and 10 is high

Add these numbers to your monthly review graph

P.S. You can do this!

END OF WEEK REVIEW

Symptom.........................
M T W T F S S
Weekly Average*

Symptom.........................
M T W T F S S
Weekly Average*

Symptom.........................
M T W T F S S
Weekly Average*

Symptom.........................
M T W T F S S
Weekly Average*

Symptom.........................
M T W T F S S
Weekly Average*

Remember to add Monday to Sunday rating onto your graph on the monthly review page

And add the weekly average to your 3 month graph at the start of this book.

Meds I took this week:

Achievements

Challenges faced

Things to order (medication/equipment/etc)

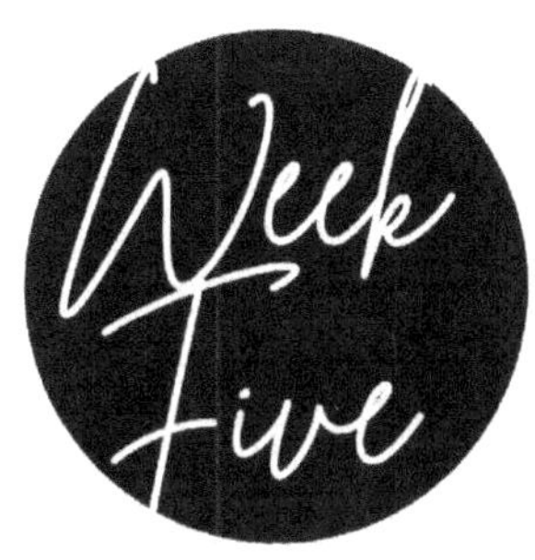

Let's get stuck in to week 5 warrior!

Check through the whole weeks sheets before
starting so you don't miss anything

Quote for the week:

Things in life will make you bitter or make you better.
You choose which one is the outcome

PILL / SUPPLEMENT TRACKER

key:

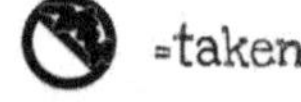

Use different colours for different medications

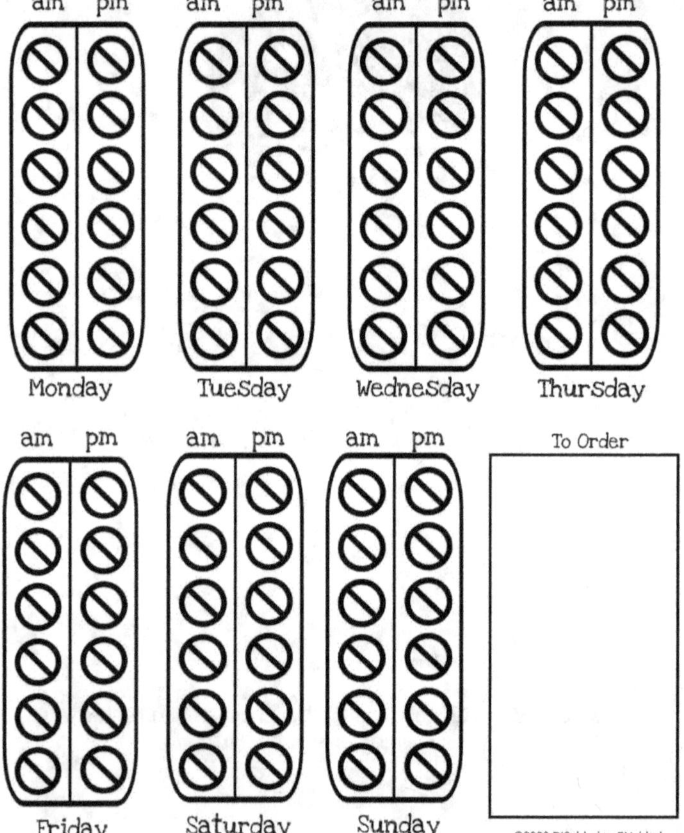

"I can handle anything"

TREATMENT DIARY

Treatment ____________________ Start date: __________

Date	Dose	pre/post meds taken	Reactions/ side effects	My treat will be

"What doesn't challenge us, doesn't change us"
You can do this.

TREATMENT DIARY

Treatment ______________________ Start date: ____________

Date	Dose	pre/post meds taken	Reactions/ side effects	My treat will be

"What doesn't challenge us, doesn't change us"
You can do this.

FOOD DIARY

	Monday	Tuesday	Wednesday	Thursday	Friday	Saturday	Sunday
Breakfast							
Snacks							
Lunch							
Snacks							
Dinner							
Snacks							

HYDRATION TRACKER

Grab a big bottle of water and add the amount of water you've drank in a day.

M	T	W	T	F	S	S

DAILY CHECK IN

Date:...

DAILY 'I AM'S'

Keep them positive! E.g. 'I am able to do anything'

I AM...

I AM...

I AM...

I AM...

I AM...

GRATEFULNESS

Today I am grateful for...

TODAY'S PRIORITIES:

★

★

★

JOURNAL SPACE: What is on your mind today?

SYMPTOMS I FEEL TODAY

Rate each symptom in severity from 1-10. 1 being low and 10 is high

Add these numbers to your monthly review graph

P.S. You can do this!

DAILY CHECK IN

Date:..

DAILY 'I AM'S'

Keep them positive! E.g. 'I am able to do anything'

I AM...

I AM...

I AM...

I AM...

I AM...

GRATEFULNESS

Today I am grateful for...

TODAY'S PRIORITIES:

★

★

★

JOURNAL SPACE: What is on your mind today?

SYMPTOMS I FEEL TODAY

Rate each Symptom in Severity from 1-10. 1 being low and 10 is high

Add these numbers to your monthly review graph

P.S. You can do this!

DAILY CHECK IN

Date:..

DAILY 'I AM'S'

Keep them positive! E.g. 'I am able to do anything'

I AM...

I AM...

I AM...

I AM...

I AM...

GRATEFULNESS

Today I am grateful for...

TODAY'S PRIORITIES:

★

★

★

JOURNAL SPACE: What is on your mind today?

SYMPTOMS I FEEL TODAY

Rate each symptom in severity from 1-10. 1 being low and 10 is high

Add these numbers to your monthly review graph

P.S. You can do this!

DAILY CHECK IN

Date:...

DAILY 'I AM'S'

Keep them positive! E.g. 'I am able to do anything'

I AM...

I AM...

I AM...

I AM...

I AM...

GRATEFULNESS

Today I am grateful for...

TODAY'S PRIORITIES:

★

★

★

JOURNAL SPACE: What is on your mind today?

SYMPTOMS I FEEL TODAY

Rate each symptom in severity from 1-10. 1 being low and 10 is high

Add these numbers to your monthly review graph

P.S. You can do this!

DAILY CHECK IN

Date:..

DAILY 'I AM'S'

Keep them positive! E.g. 'I am able to do anything'

I AM...

I AM...

I AM...

I AM...

I AM...

GRATEFULNESS

Today I am grateful for...

TODAY'S PRIORITIES:

★

★

★

JOURNAL SPACE: What is on your mind today?

SYMPTOMS I FEEL TODAY

Rate each symptom in severity from 1-10. 1 being low and 10 is high

Add these numbers to your monthly review graph

P.S. You can do this!

DAILY CHECK IN

Date:...

DAILY 'I AM'S'

Keep them positive! E.g. 'I am able to do anything'

I AM...

I AM...

I AM...

I AM...

I AM...

GRATEFULNESS

Today I am grateful for...

TODAY'S PRIORITIES:

★

★

★

JOURNAL SPACE: What is on your mind today?

SYMPTOMS I FEEL TODAY

Rate each symptom in severity from 1-10. 1 being low and 10 is high

Add these numbers to your monthly review graph

P.S. You can do this!

DAILY CHECK IN

Date:..

DAILY 'I AM'S'

Keep them positive! E.g. 'I am able to do anything'

I AM...

I AM...

I AM...

I AM...

I AM...

GRATEFULNESS

Today I am grateful for...

TODAY'S PRIORITIES:

★

★

★

JOURNAL SPACE: What is on your mind today?

SYMPTOMS I FEEL TODAY

Rate each symptom in severity from 1-10. 1 being low and 10 is high

Add these numbers to your monthly review graph

P.S. You can do this!

END OF WEEK REVIEW

Symptom........................

M T W T F S S

Weekly Average*

Symptom........................

M T W T F S S

Weekly Average*

Symptom........................

M T W T F S S

Weekly Average*

Symptom........................

M T W T F S S

Weekly Average*

Symptom........................

M T W T F S S

Weekly Average*

Remember to add Monday to Sunday rating onto your graph on the monthly review page

And add the weekly average to your 3 month graph at the start of this book.

Meds I took this week:

Achievements

Challenges faced

Things to order (medication/equipment/etc)

END OF MONTH REVIEW

Achievements

Challenges faced

Things to order (medication/equipment/etc)

Goal for this month was:

Things to focus on next month

Progress

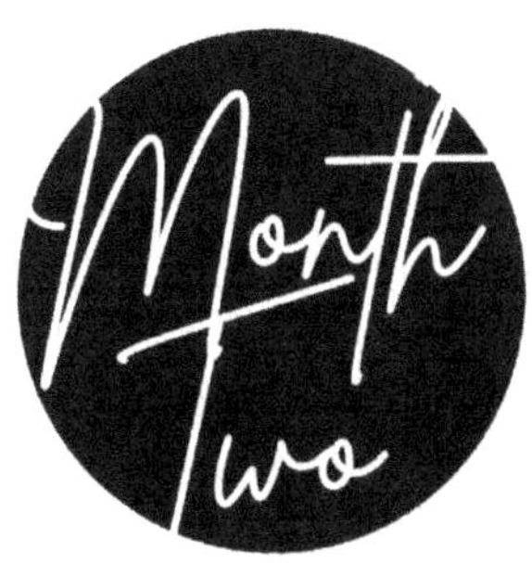

You are doing so well warrior, hang in there.

Now's the time to start fresh.
Get a new perspective.
Set new goals.
Refresh and renew.

What's your word of the month that represents what you're focussing on?

My word for this month is...

CALENDAR

Month: ....

M	T	W	T	F	S	S

I need to remember:

APPOINTMENT TRACKER

Appointment with:

On:

At:

My treat after will be:

Remember

- [ ]
- [ ]
- [ ]
- [ ]
- [ ]

Remember to ask/tell them about:

They said:

APPOINTMENT TRACKER

Appointment with:

On:

At:

My treat after will be:

Remember

- [ ]
- [ ]
- [ ]
- [ ]
- [ ]

Remember to ask/tell them about:

They said:

APPOINTMENT TRACKER

Appointment with:

On:

At:

My treat after will be:

Remember

- [ ]
- [ ]
- [ ]
- [ ]
- [ ]

Remember to ask/tell them about:

They said:

APPOINTMENT TRACKER

Appointment with:

On:

At:

My treat after will be:

Remember

- [ ]
- [ ]
- [ ]
- [ ]
- [ ]

Remember to ask/tell them about:

They said:

1 MONTH REVIEW

Take the numbers from your daily sheets and plot them on
this graph to help your medical professional get a quick glance of your health

Dates from and to: ______________________________

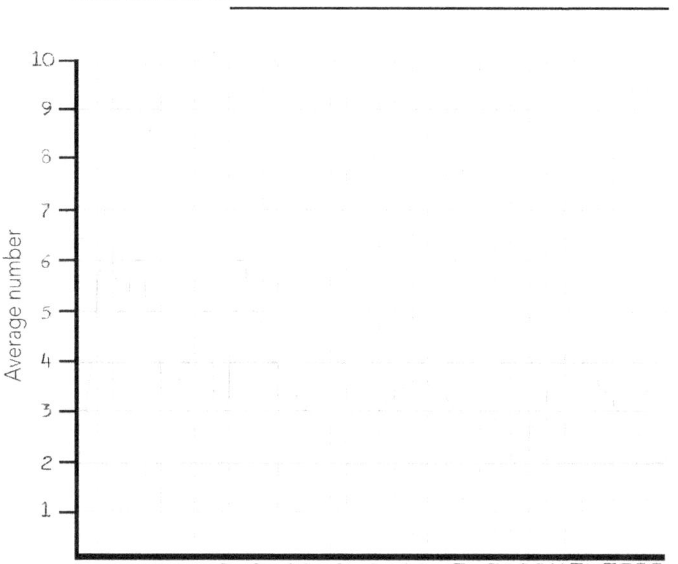

Make a note of the date under the day

Key (use a different colour line for each symptom)

Line	Symptom

Key points to discuss

You have a 100% track record for survivng the bad times, that's pretty good going!

EXERCISE TRACKER

Track your exercise progress in each of the boxes, write the activity that you did.
Make sure to write in your goal at the bottom!

Start

Finish

My goal is:

MENSTRUAL TRACKER

Month..

Key = ◩ = Normal Flow ■ = Heavy Flow ⊡ = Spotting

M	T	W	T	F	S	S

Add the calendar dates into the boxes of the month so you can see any patterns between symptoms

GOAL TRACKER

Have goals you want to complete this month? This is for you.
Add your goals to the bottom of the page so you can work backwards to work out what you need to do to reach that goal

Start

Finish

My goals are:

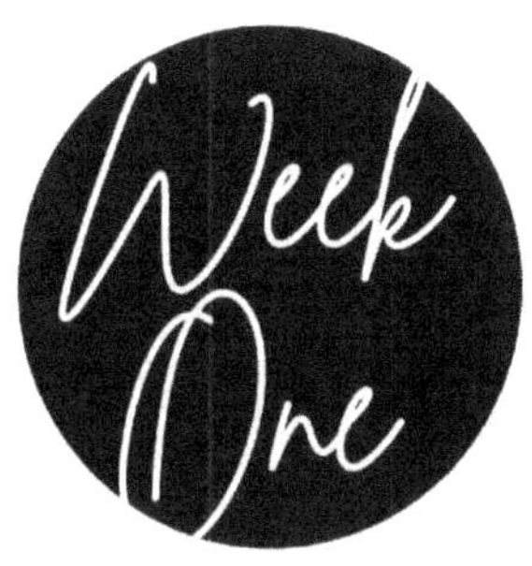

Let's get stuck in to week 1 warrior!

Check through the whole weeks sheets before starting so you don't miss anything

Quote for the week:

You can't worry about something that you have no control over.

PILL / SUPPLEMENT TRACKER

key:

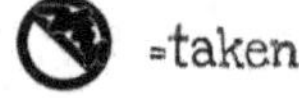

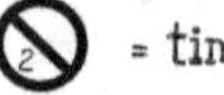

Use different colours for different medications

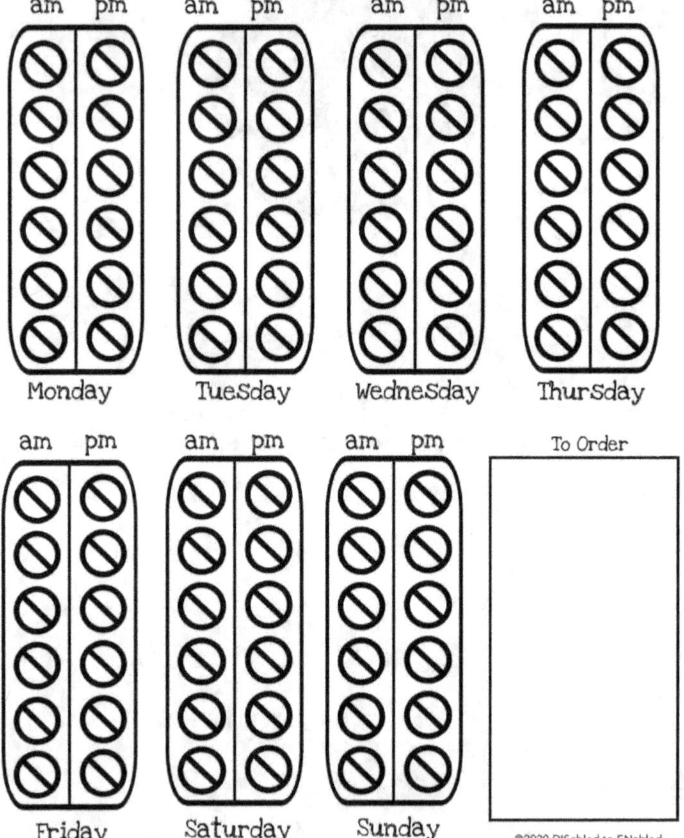

"I can handle anything"

TREATMENT DIARY

Treatment ____________________ Start date: __________

Date	Dose	pre/post meds taken	Reactions/ side effects	My treat will be

"What doesn't challenge us, doesn't change us"
You can do this.

TREATMENT DIARY

Treatment ____________________ Start date: __________

Date	Dose	pre/post meds taken	Reactions/ side effects	My treat will be

"What doesn't challenge us, doesn't change us"
You can do this.

FOOD DIARY

	Monday	Tuesday	Wednesday	Thursday	Friday	Saturday	Sunday
Breakfast							
Snacks							
Lunch							
Snacks							
Dinner							
Snacks							

HYDRATION TRACKER

Grab a big bottle of water and add the amount of water you've drank in a day.

M	T	W	T	F	S	S

DAILY CHECK IN

Date:..

DAILY 'I AM'S'

Keep them positive! E.g. 'I am able to do anything'

I AM...

I AM...

I AM...

I AM...

I AM...

TODAY'S PRIORITIES:

★

★

★

GRATEFULNESS

Today I am grateful for...

JOURNAL SPACE: What is on your mind today?

SYMPTOMS I FEEL TODAY

Rate each symptom in severity from 1-10. 1 being low and 10 is high

Add these numbers to your monthly review graph

P.S. You can do this!

DAILY CHECK IN

Date:..

DAILY 'I AM'S'

Keep them positive! E.g. 'I am able to do anything'

I AM...

I AM...

I AM...

I AM...

I AM...

GRATEFULNESS

Today I am grateful for...

TODAY'S PRIORITIES:

★

★

★

JOURNAL SPACE: What is on your mind today?

SYMPTOMS I FEEL TODAY

Rate each symptom in severity from 1-10. 1 being low and 10 is high

Add these numbers to your monthly review graph

P.S. You can do this!

DAILY CHECK IN

Date:.......................................

DAILY 'I AM'S'

Keep them positive! E.g. 'I am able to do anything'

I AM...

I AM...

I AM...

I AM...

I AM...

GRATEFULNESS

Today I am grateful for...

TODAY'S PRIORITIES:

★

★

★

JOURNAL SPACE: What is on your mind today?

SYMPTOMS I FEEL TODAY

Rate each symptom in severity from 1-10. 1 being low and 10 is high

Add these numbers to your monthly review graph

P.S. You can do this!

DAILY CHECK IN Date:..

DAILY 'I AM'S'

Keep them positive! E.g. 'I am able to do anything'

I AM...

I AM...

I AM...

I AM...

I AM...

GRATEFULNESS

Today I am grateful for...

TODAY'S PRIORITIES:

★

★

★

JOURNAL SPACE: What is on your mind today?

SYMPTOMS I FEEL TODAY

Rate each symptom in severity from 1-10 1 being low and 10 is high

Add these numbers to your monthly review graph

P.S. You can do this!

DAILY CHECK IN

Date:..

DAILY 'I AM'S'

Keep them positive! E.g. 'I am able to do anything'

I AM...

I AM...

I AM...

I AM...

I AM...

GRATEFULNESS

Today I am grateful for...

TODAY'S PRIORITIES:

★

★

★

JOURNAL SPACE: What is on your mind today?

SYMPTOMS I FEEL TODAY

Rate each symptom in severity from 1-10. 1 being low and 10 is high

Add these numbers to your monthly review graph

P.S. You can do this!

DAILY CHECK IN

Date:..

DAILY 'I AM'S'

Keep them positive! E.g. 'I am able to do anything'

I AM...

I AM...

I AM...

I AM...

I AM...

GRATEFULNESS

Today I am grateful for...

TODAY'S PRIORITIES:

★

★

★

JOURNAL SPACE: What is on your mind today?

SYMPTOMS I FEEL TODAY

Rate each symptom in severity from 1-10. 1 being low and 10 is high

Add these numbers to your monthly review graph

P.S. You can do this!

DAILY CHECK IN

Date:..

DAILY 'I AM'S'

Keep them positive! E.g. 'I am able to do anything'

I AM...

I AM...

I AM...

I AM...

I AM...

GRATEFULNESS

Today I am grateful for...

TODAY'S PRIORITIES:

★

★

★

JOURNAL SPACE: What is on your mind today?

SYMPTOMS I FEEL TODAY

Rate each symptom in severity from 1-10. 1 being low and 10 is high

Add these numbers to your monthly review graph

P.S. You can do this!

END OF WEEK REVIEW

Symptom.......................

M	T	W	T	F	S	S	Weekly Average*

Symptom.......................

M	T	W	T	F	S	S	Weekly Average*

Symptom.......................

M	T	W	T	F	S	S	Weekly Average*

Symptom.......................

M	T	W	T	F	S	S	Weekly Average*

Symptom.......................

M	T	W	T	F	S	S	Weekly Average*

Remember to add Monday to Sunday rating onto your graph on the monthly review page

And add the weekly average to your 3 month graph at the start of this book.

Meds I took this week:

Achievements

Challenges faced

Things to order (medication/equipment/etc)

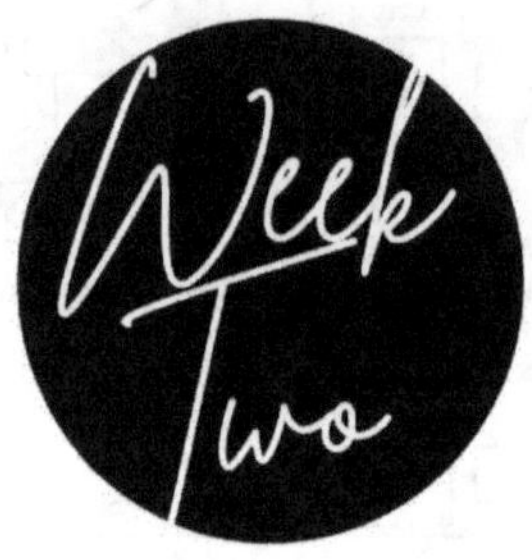

These are your pages to be filled in after a week.

You'll find a medication sheet, timetable, food diary, mood tracker, sleep tracker and dream diary.

These sheets combined keep you organised and in control.

Use these sheets for creating patterns between different things.

Tip: Fill in daily if you think you may not remember, otherwise fill this in on a Sunday eve to be ready for the next week.

PILL / SUPPLEMENT TRACKER

key:

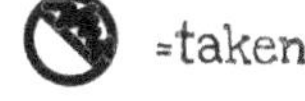
=taken

= time

Use different colours for different medications

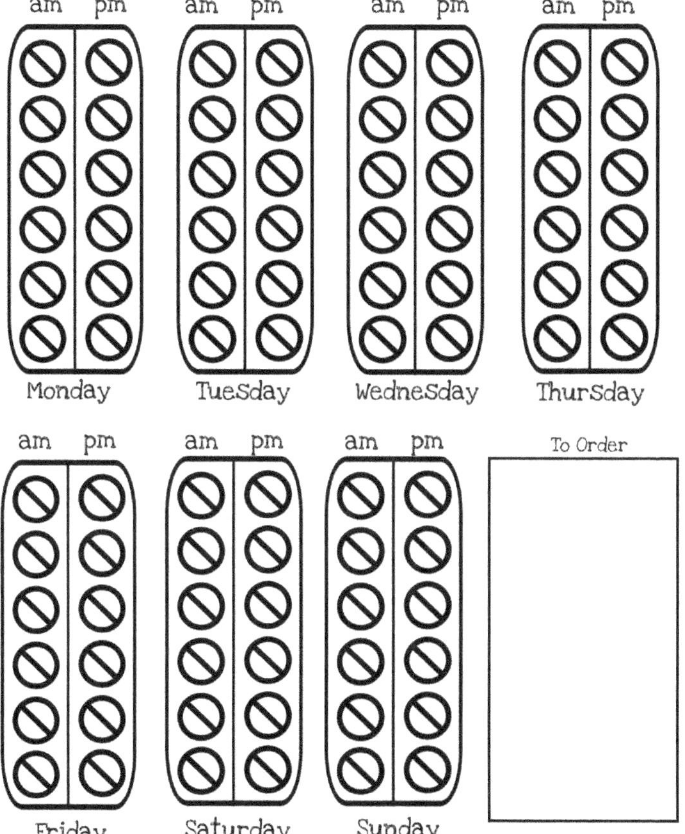

"I can handle anything"

TREATMENT DIARY

Treatment ____________________ Start date: __________

Date	Dose	pre/post meds taken	Reactions/ side effects	My treat will be

"What doesn't challenge us, doesn't change us"
You can do this.

TREATMENT DIARY

Treatment ____________________ Start date: __________

Date	Dose	pre/post meds taken	Reactions/ side effects	My treat will be

"What doesn't challenge us, doesn't change us"
You can do this.

FOOD DIARY

	Monday	Tuesday	Wednesday	Thursday	Friday	Saturday	Sunday
Breakfast							
Snacks							
Lunch							
Snacks							
Dinner							
Snacks							

HYDRATION TRACKER

Grab a big bottle of water and add the amount of water you've drank in a day.

M	T	W	T	F	S	S

DAILY CHECK IN

Date:..

DAILY 'I AM'S'

Keep them positive! E.g. 'I am able to do anything'

I AM...

I AM...

I AM...

I AM...

I AM...

GRATEFULNESS

Today I am grateful for...

TODAY'S PRIORITIES:

★

★

★

JOURNAL SPACE: What is on your mind today?

SYMPTOMS I FEEL TODAY

Rate each symptom in severity from 1-10. 1 being low and 10 is high

Add these numbers to your monthly review graph

P.S. You can do this!

DAILY CHECK IN

Date:..

DAILY 'I AM'S'

Keep them positive! E.g. 'I am able to do anything'

I AM...

I AM...

I AM...

I AM...

I AM...

GRATEFULNESS

Today I am grateful for...

TODAY'S PRIORITIES:

★

★

★

JOURNAL SPACE: What is on your mind today?

SYMPTOMS I FEEL TODAY

Rate each symptom in severity from 1-10. 1 being low and 10 is high

Add these numbers to your monthly review graph

P.S. You can do this!

DAILY CHECK IN

Date:..

DAILY 'I AM'S'

Keep them positive! E.g. 'I am able to do anything'

I AM...

I AM...

I AM...

I AM...

I AM...

GRATEFULNESS

Today I am grateful for...

TODAY'S PRIORITIES:

★

★

★

JOURNAL SPACE: What is on your mind today?

SYMPTOMS I FEEL TODAY

Rate each symptom in severity from 1-10 1 being low and 10 is high

Add these numbers to your monthly review graph

P.S. You can do this!

DAILY CHECK IN

Date:...

DAILY 'I AM'S'

Keep them positive! E.g. 'I am able to do anything'

I AM...

I AM...

I AM...

I AM...

I AM...

TODAY'S PRIORITIES:

★

★

★

GRATEFULNESS

Today I am grateful for...

JOURNAL SPACE: What is on your mind today?

SYMPTOMS I FEEL TODAY

Rate each symptom in severity from 1-10. 1 being low and 10 is high

Add these numbers to your monthly review graph

P.S. You can do this!

DAILY CHECK IN

Date:

DAILY 'I AM'S'

Keep them positive! E.g. 'I am able to do anything'

I AM...

I AM...

I AM...

I AM...

I AM...

TODAY'S PRIORITIES:

★

★

★

GRATEFULNESS

Today I am grateful for...

JOURNAL SPACE: What is on your mind today?

SYMPTOMS I FEEL TODAY

Rate each symptom in severity from 1-10. 1 being low and 10 is high

Add these numbers to your monthly review graph

P.S. You can do this!

DAILY CHECK IN

Date:...

DAILY 'I AM'S'

Keep them positive! E.g. 'I am able to do anything'

I AM...

I AM...

I AM...

I AM...

I AM...

GRATEFULNESS

Today I am grateful for...

TODAY'S PRIORITIES:

★

★

★

JOURNAL SPACE: What is on your mind today?

SYMPTOMS I FEEL TODAY

Rate each symptom in severity from 1-10. 1 being low and 10 is high

Add these numbers to your monthly review graph

P.S. You can do this!

DAILY CHECK IN

Date:...

DAILY 'I AM'S'

Keep them positive! E.g. 'I am able to do anything'

I AM...

I AM...

I AM...

I AM...

I AM...

GRATEFULNESS

Today I am grateful for...

TODAY'S PRIORITIES:

★

★

★

JOURNAL SPACE: What is on your mind today?

SYMPTOMS I FEEL TODAY

Rate each Symptom in severity from 1-10. 1 being low and 10 is high

Add these numbers to your monthly review graph

P.S. You can do this!

END OF WEEK REVIEW

Symptom.......................
M T W T F S S
Weekly Average*

Symptom.......................
M T W T F S S
Weekly Average*

Symptom.......................
M T W T F S S
Weekly Average*

Symptom.......................
M T W T F S S
Weekly Average*

Symptom.......................
M T W T F S S
Weekly Average*

Remember to add Monday to Sunday rating onto your graph on the monthly review page

And add the weekly average to your 3 month graph at the start of this book.

Meds I took this week:

Achievements

Challenges faced

Things to order (medication/equipment/etc)

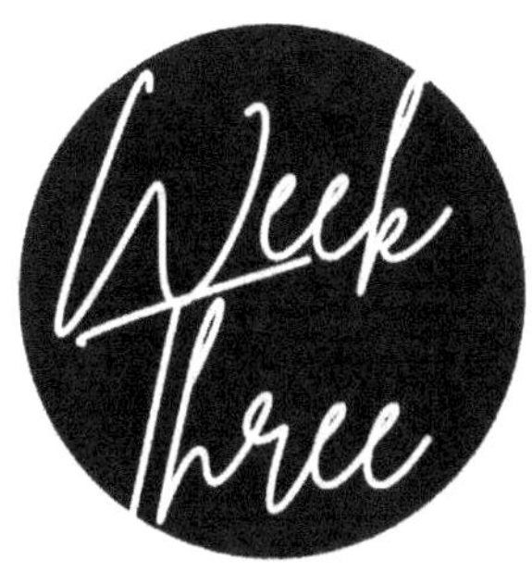

Let's get stuck in to week 3 warrior!

Check through the whole weeks sheets before starting so you don't miss anything

Quote for the week:

How would the person I want to be, do the things that I want to do now?

PILL / SUPPLEMENT TRACKER

key:

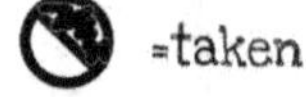
=taken

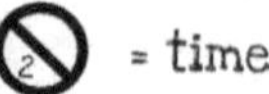
= time

Use different colours for different medications

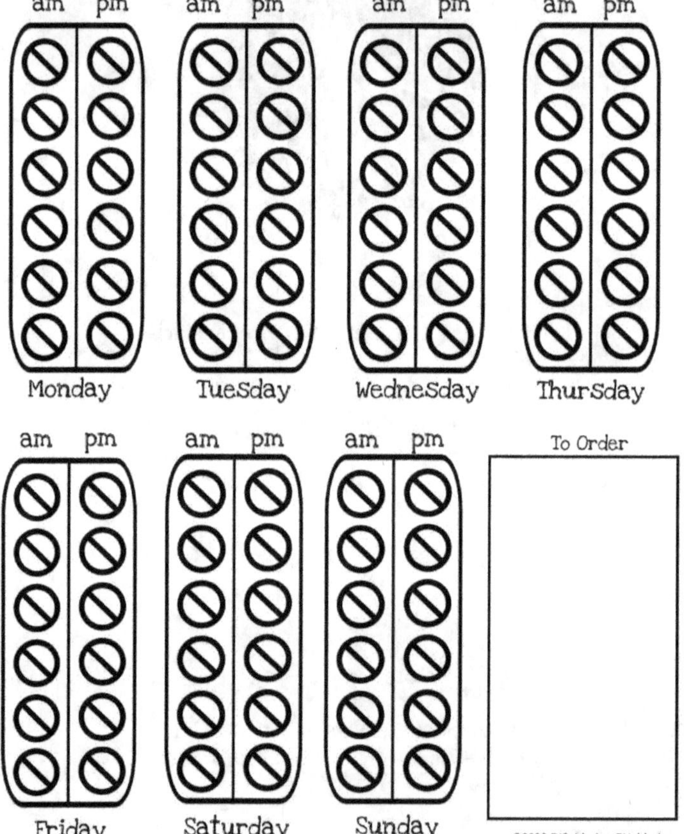

To Order

"I can handle anything"

TREATMENT DIARY

Treatment ____________________ Start date: __________

Date	Dose	pre/post meds taken	Reactions/ side effects	My treat will be

"What doesn't challenge us, doesn't change us"
You can do this.

TREATMENT DIARY

Treatment ____________________ Start date: __________

Date	Dose	pre/post meds taken	Reactions/ side effects	My treat will be

"What doesn't challenge us, doesn't change us"
You can do this.

FOOD DIARY

	Monday	Tuesday	Wednesday	Thursday	Friday	Saturday	Sunday
Breakfast							
Snacks							
Lunch							
Snacks							
Dinner							
Snacks							

HYDRATION TRACKER

Grab a big bottle of water and add the amount of water you've drank in a day.

M	T	W	T	F	S	S

DAILY CHECK IN

Date:..

DAILY 'I AM'S'

Keep them positive! E.g. 'I am able to do anything'

I AM...

I AM...

I AM...

I AM...

I AM...

GRATEFULNESS

Today I am grateful for...

TODAY'S PRIORITIES:

★

★

★

JOURNAL SPACE: What is on your mind today?

SYMPTOMS I FEEL TODAY

Rate each symptom in severity from 1-10. 1 being low and 10 is high

Add these numbers to your monthly review graph

P.S. You can do this!

DAILY CHECK IN

Date:..

DAILY 'I AM'S'

Keep them positive! E.g. 'I am able to do anything'

I AM...

I AM...

I AM...

I AM...

I AM...

TODAY'S PRIORITIES:

★

★

★

GRATEFULNESS

Today I am grateful for...

JOURNAL SPACE: What is on your mind today?

SYMPTOMS I FEEL TODAY

Rate each symptom in severity from 1-10. 1 being low and 10 is high

Add these numbers to your monthly review graph

P.S. You can do this!

DAILY CHECK IN

Date:..

DAILY 'I AM'S'

Keep them positive! E.g. 'I am able to do anything'

I AM...

I AM...

I AM...

I AM...

I AM...

GRATEFULNESS

Today I am grateful for...

TODAY'S PRIORITIES:

★

★

★

JOURNAL SPACE: What is on your mind today?

SYMPTOMS I FEEL TODAY

Rate each symptom in severity from 1-10. 1 being low and 10 is high

Add these numbers to your monthly review graph

P.S. You can do this!

DAILY CHECK IN

Date:..

DAILY 'I AM'S'

Keep them positive! E.g. 'I am able to do anything'

I AM...

I AM...

I AM...

I AM...

I AM...

GRATEFULNESS

Today I am grateful for...

TODAY'S PRIORITIES:

★

★

★

JOURNAL SPACE: What is on your mind today?

SYMPTOMS I FEEL TODAY

Rate each symptom in severity from 1-10. 1 being low and 10 is high

Add these numbers to your monthly review graph

P.S. You can do this!

DAILY CHECK IN

Date:...

DAILY 'I AM'S'

Keep them positive! E.g. 'I am able to do anything'

I AM...

I AM...

I AM...

I AM...

I AM...

GRATEFULNESS

Today I am grateful for...

TODAY'S PRIORITIES:

★

★

★

JOURNAL SPACE: What is on your mind today?

SYMPTOMS I FEEL TODAY

Rate each symptom in severity from 1-10. 1 being low and 10 is high

Add these numbers to your monthly review graph

P.S. You can do this!

DAILY CHECK IN

Date:..

DAILY 'I AM'S'

Keep them positive! E.g. 'I am able to do anything'

I AM...

I AM...

I AM...

I AM...

I AM...

GRATEFULNESS

Today I am grateful for...

TODAY'S PRIORITIES:

★

★

★

JOURNAL SPACE: What is on your mind today?

SYMPTOMS I FEEL TODAY

Rate each symptom in severity from 1-10. 1 being low and 10 is high

Add these numbers to your monthly review graph

P.S. You can do this!

DAILY CHECK IN

Date:..

DAILY 'I AM'S'

Keep them positive! E.g. 'I am able to do anything'

I AM...

I AM...

I AM...

I AM...

I AM...

GRATEFULNESS

Today I am grateful for...

TODAY'S PRIORITIES:

★

★

★

JOURNAL SPACE: What is on your mind today?

SYMPTOMS I FEEL TODAY

Rate each symptom in severity from 1-10. 1 being low and 10 is high

Add these numbers to your monthly review graph

P.S. You can do this!

END OF WEEK REVIEW

Symptom........................

M	T	W	T	F	S	S	Weekly Average*

Symptom........................

M	T	W	T	F	S	S	Weekly Average*

Symptom........................

M	T	W	T	F	S	S	Weekly Average*

Symptom........................

M	T	W	T	F	S	S	Weekly Average*

Symptom........................

M	T	W	T	F	S	S	Weekly Average*

Remember to add Monday to Sunday rating onto your graph on the monthly review page

And add the weekly average to your 3 month graph at the start of this book

Meds I took this week:

Achievements

Challenges faced

Things to order (medication/equipment/etc)

Let's get stuck in to week 4 warrior!

Check through the whole weeks sheets before starting so you don't miss anything

Quote for the week:

As long as you breathe you got a shot at your dream.

PILL / SUPPLEMENT TRACKER

key:

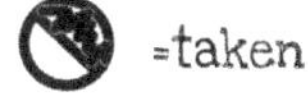
=taken

= time

Use different colours for different medications

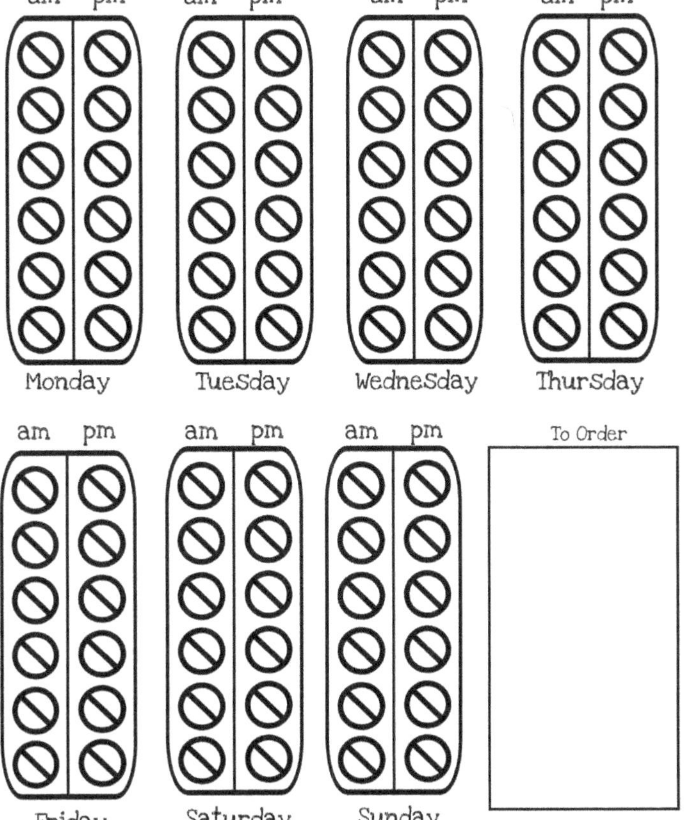

"I can handle anything"

TREATMENT DIARY

Treatment ______________________ Start date: ____________

Date	Dose	pre/post meds taken	Reactions/ side effects	My treat will be

"What doesn't challenge us, doesn't change us"
You can do this.

TREATMENT DIARY

Treatment ____________________ Start date: __________

Date	Dose	pre/post meds taken	Reactions/ side effects	My treat will be

"What doesn't challenge us, doesn't change us"
You can do this.

FOOD DIARY

	Monday	Tuesday	Wednesday	Thursday	Friday	Saturday	Sunday
Breakfast							
Snacks							
Lunch							
Snacks							
Dinner							
Snacks							

HYDRATION TRACKER

Grab a big bottle of water and add the amount of water you've drank in a day.

M	T	W	T	F	S	S

DAILY CHECK IN

Date:..

DAILY 'I AM'S'

Keep them positive! E.g. 'I am able to do anything'

I AM...

I AM...

I AM...

I AM...

I AM...

TODAY'S PRIORITIES:

★

★

★

GRATEFULNESS

Today I am grateful for...

JOURNAL SPACE: What is on your mind today?

SYMPTOMS I FEEL TODAY

Rate each symptom in severity from 1-10. 1 being low and 10 is high

Add these numbers to your monthly review graph

P.S. You can do this!

DAILY CHECK IN

Date:..

DAILY 'I AM'S'

Keep them positive! E.g. 'I am able to do anything'

I AM...

I AM...

I AM...

I AM...

I AM...

GRATEFULNESS

Today I am grateful for...

TODAY'S PRIORITIES:

★

★

★

JOURNAL SPACE: What is on your mind today?

SYMPTOMS I FEEL TODAY

Rate each symptom in severity from 1-10. 1 being low and 10 is high

Add these numbers to your monthly review graph

P.S. You can do this!

DAILY CHECK IN

Date:..

DAILY 'I AM'S'

Keep them positive! E.g. 'I am able to do anything'

I AM...

I AM...

I AM...

I AM...

I AM...

GRATEFULNESS

Today I am grateful for...

TODAY'S PRIORITIES:

★

★

★

JOURNAL SPACE: What is on your mind today?

SYMPTOMS I FEEL TODAY

Rate each symptom in severity from 1-10. 1 being low and 10 is high

Add these numbers to your monthly review graph

P.S. You can do this!

DAILY CHECK IN

Date:...

DAILY 'I AM'S'

Keep them positive! E.g. 'I am able to do anything'

I AM...

I AM...

I AM...

I AM...

I AM...

GRATEFULNESS

Today I am grateful for...

TODAY'S PRIORITIES:

★

★

★

JOURNAL SPACE: What is on your mind today?

SYMPTOMS I FEEL TODAY

Rate each symptom in severity from 1-10. 1 being low and 10 is high

Add these numbers to your monthly review graph

P.S. You can do this!

DAILY CHECK IN

Date:..

DAILY 'I AM'S'

Keep them positive! E.g. 'I am able to do anything'

I AM...

I AM...

I AM...

I AM...

I AM...

GRATEFULNESS

Today I am grateful for...

TODAY'S PRIORITIES:

★

★

★

JOURNAL SPACE: What is on your mind today?

SYMPTOMS I FEEL TODAY

Rate each symptom in severity from 1-10: 1 being low and 10 is high

Add these numbers to your monthly review graph

P.S. You can do this!

DAILY CHECK IN

Date:..

DAILY 'I AM'S'

Keep them positive! E.g. 'I am able to do anything'

I AM...

I AM...

I AM...

I AM...

I AM...

GRATEFULNESS

Today I am grateful for...

TODAY'S PRIORITIES:

★

★

★

JOURNAL SPACE: What is on your mind today?

SYMPTOMS I FEEL TODAY

Rate each symptom in severity from 1-10. 1 being low and 10 is high

Add these numbers to your monthly review graph

P.S. You can do this!

DAILY CHECK IN

Date:..

DAILY 'I AM'S'

Keep them positive! E.g. 'I am able to do anything'

I AM...

I AM...

I AM...

I AM...

I AM...

GRATEFULNESS

Today I am grateful for...

TODAY'S PRIORITIES:

★

★

★

JOURNAL SPACE: What is on your mind today?

SYMPTOMS I FEEL TODAY

Rate each symptom in severity from 1-10. 1 being low and 10 is high

Add these numbers to your monthly review graph

P.S. You can do this!

END OF WEEK REVIEW

Symptom.......................

M T W T F S S

Weekly Average*

Symptom.......................

M T W T F S S

Weekly Average*

Symptom.......................

M T W T F S S

Weekly Average*

Symptom.......................

M T W T F S S

Weekly Average*

Symptom.......................

M T W T F S S

Weekly Average*

Remember to add Monday to Sunday rating onto your graph on the monthly review page

And add the weekly average to your 3 month graph at the start of this book.

Meds I took this week:

Achievements

Challenges faced

Things to order (medication/equipment/etc)

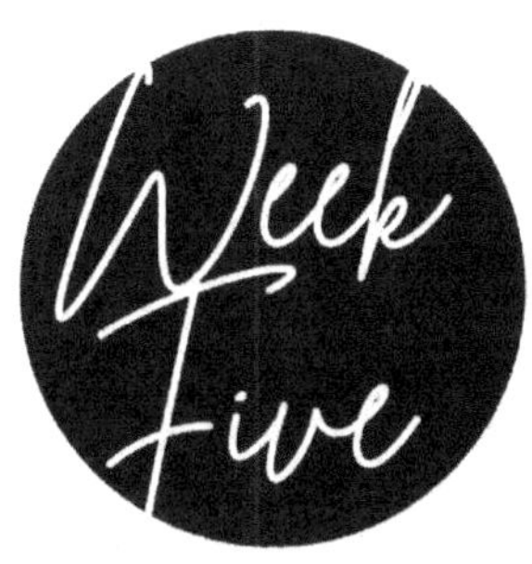

Let's get stuck in to week 5 warrior!

Check through the whole weeks sheets before
starting so you don't miss anything

Quote for the week:

Things in life will make you bitter or make you better.
You choose which one is the outcome

PILL / SUPPLEMENT TRACKER

key:

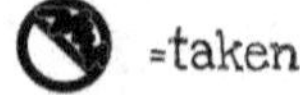 =taken

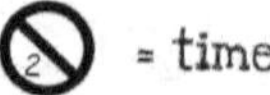 = time

Use different colours for different medications

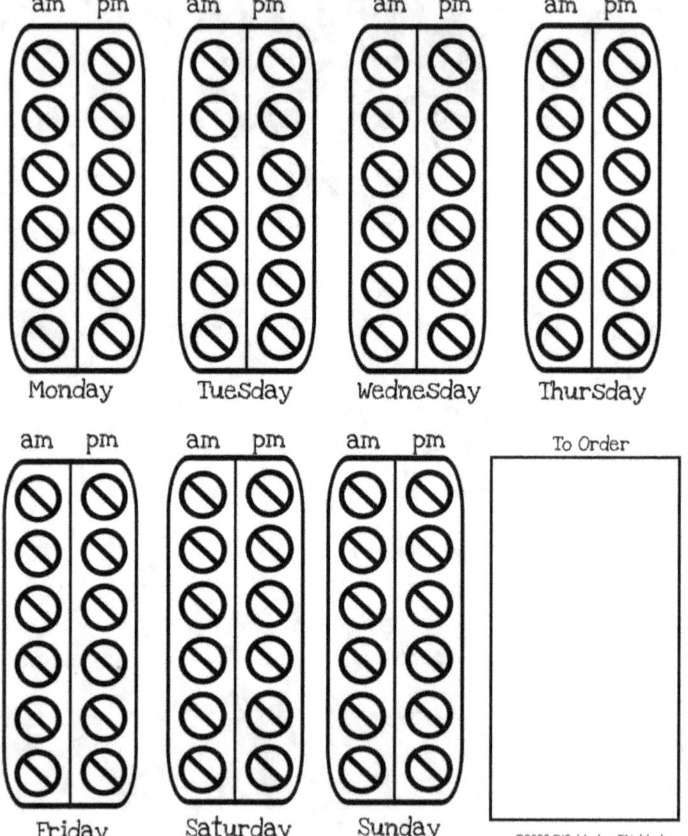

"I can handle anything"

TREATMENT DIARY

Treatment ____________________ Start date: __________

Date	Dose	pre/post meds taken	Reactions/ side effects	My treat will be

"What doesn't challenge us, doesn't change us"
You can do this.

TREATMENT DIARY

Treatment ____________________ Start date: __________

Date	Dose	pre/post meds taken	Reactions/ side effects	My treat will be

"What doesn't challenge us, doesn't change us"
You can do this.

FOOD DIARY

	Monday	Tuesday	Wednesday	Thursday	Friday	Saturday	Sunday
Breakfast							
Snacks							
Lunch							
Snacks							
Dinner							
Snacks							

HYDRATION TRACKER

Grab a big bottle of water and add the amount of water you've drank in a day.

M	T	W	T	F	S	S

DAILY CHECK IN

Date:...

DAILY 'I AM'S'

Keep them positive! E.g. 'I am able to do anything'

I AM...

I AM...

I AM...

I AM...

I AM...

GRATEFULNESS

Today I am grateful for...

TODAY'S PRIORITIES:

★

★

★

JOURNAL SPACE: What is on your mind today?

SYMPTOMS I FEEL TODAY

Rate each symptom in severity from 1-10. 1 being low and 10 is high

Add these numbers to your monthly review graph

P.S. You can do this!

DAILY CHECK IN

Date:...

DAILY 'I AM'S'

Keep them positive! E.g. 'I am able to do anything'

I AM...

I AM...

I AM...

I AM...

I AM...

GRATEFULNESS

Today I am grateful for...

TODAY'S PRIORITIES:

★

★

★

JOURNAL SPACE: What is on your mind today?

SYMPTOMS I FEEL TODAY

Rate each symptom in severity from 1-10. 1 being low and 10 is high

Add these numbers to your monthly review graph

P.S. You can do this!

DAILY CHECK IN

Date:..

DAILY 'I AM'S'

Keep them positive! E.g. 'I am able to do anything'

I AM...

I AM...

I AM...

I AM...

I AM...

GRATEFULNESS

Today I am grateful for...

TODAY'S PRIORITIES:

★

★

★

JOURNAL SPACE: What is on your mind today?

SYMPTOMS I FEEL TODAY

Rate each symptom in severity from 1-10. 1 being low and 10 is high

Add these numbers to your monthly review graph

P.S. You can do this!

DAILY CHECK IN

Date:...

DAILY 'I AM'S'

Keep them positive! E.g. 'I am able to do anything'

I AM...

I AM...

I AM...

I AM...

I AM...

GRATEFULNESS

Today I am grateful for...

TODAY'S PRIORITIES:

★

★

★

JOURNAL SPACE: What is on your mind today?

SYMPTOMS I FEEL TODAY

Rate each Symptom in severity from 1-10. 1 being low and 10 is high

Add these numbers to your monthly review graph

P.S. You can do this!

DAILY CHECK IN

Date:..

DAILY 'I AM'S'

Keep them positive! E.g. 'I am able to do anything'

I AM...

I AM...

I AM...

I AM...

I AM...

GRATEFULNESS

Today I am grateful for...

TODAY'S PRIORITIES:

★

★

★

JOURNAL SPACE: What is on your mind today?

SYMPTOMS I FEEL TODAY

Rate each symptom in severity from 1-10. 1 being low and 10 is high

Add these numbers to your monthly review graph

P.S. You can do this!

DAILY CHECK IN

Date:..

DAILY 'I AM'S'

Keep them positive! E.g. 'I am able to do anything'

I AM...

I AM...

I AM...

I AM...

I AM...

GRATEFULNESS

Today I am grateful for...

TODAY'S PRIORITIES:

★

★

★

JOURNAL SPACE: What is on your mind today?

SYMPTOMS I FEEL TODAY

Rate each symptom in severity from 1-10. 1 being low and 10 is high

Add these numbers to your monthly review graph

P.S. You can do this!

DAILY CHECK IN

Date:..

DAILY 'I AM'S'

Keep them positive! E.g. 'I am able to do anything'

I AM...

I AM...

I AM...

I AM...

I AM...

GRATEFULNESS

Today I am grateful for...

TODAY'S PRIORITIES:

★

★

★

JOURNAL SPACE: What is on your mind today?

SYMPTOMS I FEEL TODAY

Rate each symptom in severity from 1-10. 1 being low and 10 is high

Add these numbers to your monthly review graph

P.S. You can do this!

END OF WEEK REVIEW

Symptom......................

M	T	W	T	F	S	S	Weekly Average*

Symptom......................

M	T	W	T	F	S	S	Weekly Average*

Symptom......................

M	T	W	T	F	S	S	Weekly Average*

Symptom......................

M	T	W	T	F	S	S	Weekly Average*

Symptom......................

M	T	W	T	F	S	S	Weekly Average*

Remember to add Monday to Sunday rating onto your graph on the monthly review page

And add the weekly average to your 3 month graph at the start of this book

Meds I took this week:

Achievements

Challenges faced

Things to order (medication/equipment/etc)

END OF MONTH REVIEW

Achievements

Challenges faced

Things to order (medication/equipment/etc)

Goal for this month was:

Things to focus on next month

Progress

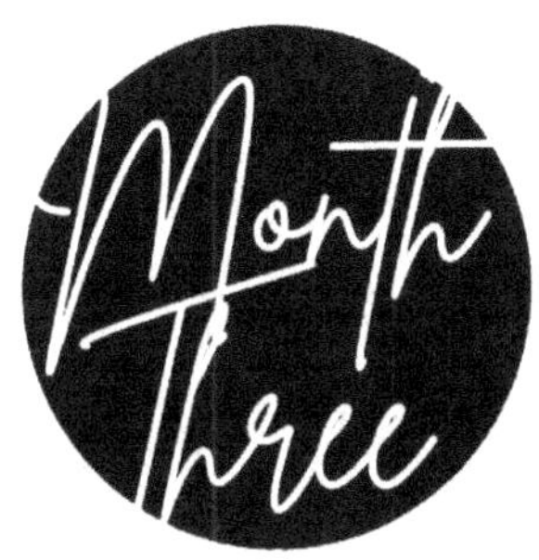

You are doing so well warrior, hang in there.

"In order to do something you've never done,
you need to become someone you've never been"
- Les Brown

You can do anything!

What's your word of the month that represents what you're focussing on?

My word for this month is

CALENDAR

Month: ....

M	T	W	T	F	S	S

I need to remember:

APPOINTMENT TRACKER

Appointment with:

On:

At:

My treat after will be:

Remember

- [ ]
- [ ]
- [ ]
- [ ]
- [ ]

Remember to ask/tell them about:

They said:

APPOINTMENT TRACKER

Appointment with:

On:

At:

My treat after will be:

Remember

- [ ]
- [ ]
- [ ]
- [ ]
- [ ]

Remember to ask/tell them about:

They said:

APPOINTMENT TRACKER

Appointment with:

On:

At:

My treat after will be:

Remember

- [ ]
- [ ]
- [ ]
- [ ]
- [ ]

Remember to ask/tell them about:

They said:

APPOINTMENT TRACKER

Appointment with:

On:

At:

My treat after will be:

Remember

☐
☐
☐
☐
☐

Remember to ask/tell them about:

They said:

1 MONTH REVIEW

Take the numbers from your daily sheets and plot them on this graph to help your medical professional get a quick glance of your health

Dates from and to: ______________________

Average number

10
9
8
7
6
5
4
3
2
1

M T W T F S S M T W T F S S M T W T F S S M T W T F S S M T W T F S S

Day

Make a note of the date under the day

Key (use a different colour line for each symptom)

Line	Symptom

Key points to discuss

You have a 100% track record for survivng the bad times, that's pretty good going!

EXERCISE TRACKER

Track your exercise progress in each of the boxes, write the activity that you did. Make sure to write in your goal at the bottom!

Start

Finish

My goal is:

MENSTRUAL TRACKER

Month..

Key = ◩ = Normal Flow ■ = Heavy Flow ⊡ = Spotting

M	T	W	T	F	S	S

Add the calendar dates into the boxes of the month so you can see any patterns between symptoms

GOAL TRACKER

Have goals you want to complete this month? This is for you.
Add your goals to the bottom of the page so you can work backwards to work out what you need to do to reach that goal

Start

Finish

My goals are:

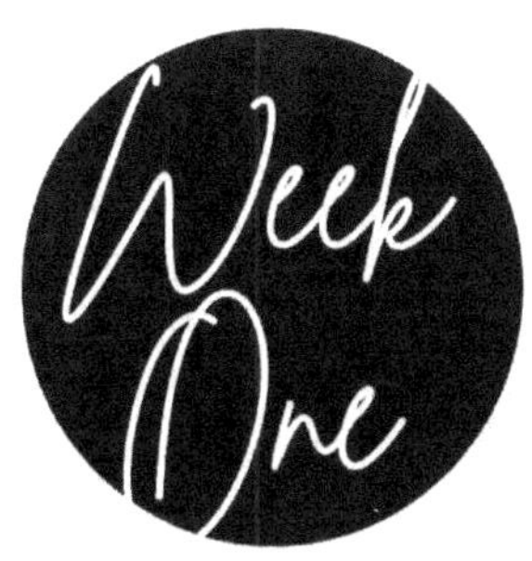

Let's get stuck in to week 1 warrior!

Check through the whole weeks sheets before starting so you don't miss anything

Quote for the week:

You can't worry about something that you have no control over.

PILL / SUPPLEMENT TRACKER

key:

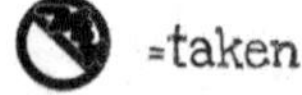
=taken

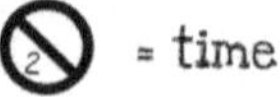
= time

Use different colours for different medications

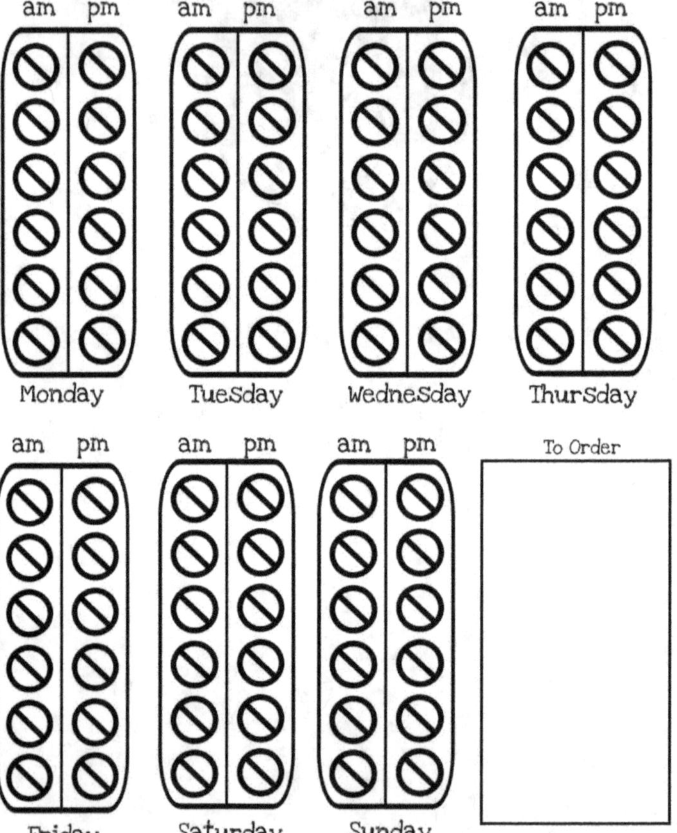

To Order

"I can handle anything"

TREATMENT DIARY

Treatment ______________________ Start date: ___________

Date	Dose	pre/post meds taken	Reactions/ side effects	My treat will be

"What doesn't challenge us, doesn't change us"
You can do this.

TREATMENT DIARY

Treatment ____________________ Start date: __________

Date	Dose	pre/post meds taken	Reactions/ side effects	My treat will be

"What doesn't challenge us, doesn't change us"
You can do this.

FOOD DIARY

	Monday	Tuesday	Wednesday	Thursday	Friday	Saturday	Sunday
Breakfast							
Snacks							
Lunch							
Snacks							
Dinner							
Snacks							

HYDRATION TRACKER

Grab a big bottle of water and add the amount of water you've drank in a day.

M	T	W	T	F	S	S

DAILY CHECK IN

Date:...

DAILY 'I AM'S'

Keep them positive! E.g. 'I am able to do anything'

I AM...

I AM...

I AM...

I AM...

I AM...

GRATEFULNESS

Today I am grateful for...

TODAY'S PRIORITIES:

★

★

★

JOURNAL SPACE: What is on your mind today?

SYMPTOMS I FEEL TODAY

Rate each symptom in severity from 1-10. 1 being low and 10 is high

Add these numbers to your monthly review graph

P.S. You can do this!

DAILY CHECK IN

Date:..

DAILY 'I AM'S'

Keep them positive! E.g. 'I am able to do anything'

I AM...

I AM...

I AM...

I AM...

I AM...

GRATEFULNESS

Today I am grateful for...

TODAY'S PRIORITIES:

★

★

★

JOURNAL SPACE: What is on your mind today?

SYMPTOMS I FEEL TODAY

Rate each symptom in severity from 1-10. 1 being low and 10 is high

Add these numbers to your monthly review graph

P.S. You can do this!

DAILY CHECK IN

Date:...

DAILY 'I AM'S'

Keep them positive! E.g. 'I am able to do anything'

I AM...

I AM...

I AM...

I AM...

I AM...

GRATEFULNESS

Today I am grateful for...

TODAY'S PRIORITIES:

★

★

★

JOURNAL SPACE: What is on your mind today?

SYMPTOMS I FEEL TODAY

Rate each symptom in severity from 1-10. 1 being low and 10 is high

Add these numbers to your monthly review graph

P.S. You can do this!

DAILY CHECK IN

Date:..

DAILY 'I AM'S'

Keep them positive! E.g. 'I am able to do anything'

I AM...

I AM...

I AM...

I AM...

I AM...

GRATEFULNESS

Today I am grateful for...

TODAY'S PRIORITIES:

★

★

★

JOURNAL SPACE: What is on your mind today?

SYMPTOMS I FEEL TODAY

Rate each symptom in severity from 1-10. 1 being low and 10 is high

Add these numbers to your monthly review graph

P.S. You can do this!

DAILY CHECK IN

Date:..

DAILY 'I AM'S'

Keep them positive! E.g. 'I am able to do anything'

I AM...

I AM...

I AM...

I AM...

I AM...

GRATEFULNESS

Today I am grateful for...

TODAY'S PRIORITIES:

★

★

★

JOURNAL SPACE: What is on your mind today?

SYMPTOMS I FEEL TODAY

Rate each symptom in severity from 1-10. 1 being low and 10 is high

Add these numbers to your monthly review graph

P.S. You can do this!

DAILY CHECK IN

Date:..

DAILY 'I AM'S'

Keep them positive! E.g. 'I am able to do anything'

I AM...

I AM...

I AM...

I AM...

I AM...

GRATEFULNESS

Today I am grateful for...

TODAY'S PRIORITIES:

★

★

★

JOURNAL SPACE: What is on your mind today?

SYMPTOMS I FEEL TODAY

Rate each symptom in severity from 1-10 1 being low and 10 is high

Add these numbers to your monthly review graph

P.S. You can do this!

DAILY CHECK IN

Date:..

DAILY 'I AM'S'

Keep them positive! E.g. 'I am able to do anything'

I AM...

I AM...

I AM...

I AM...

I AM...

GRATEFULNESS

Today I am grateful for...

TODAY'S PRIORITIES:

★

★

★

JOURNAL SPACE: What is on your mind today?

SYMPTOMS I FEEL TODAY

Rate each symptom in severity from 1-10. 1 being low and 10 is high

Add these numbers to your monthly review graph

P.S. You can do this!

END OF WEEK REVIEW

Symptom.......................... Weekly Average*

M T W T F S S

Symptom.......................... Weekly Average*

M T W T F S S

Symptom.......................... Weekly Average*

M T W T F S S

Symptom.......................... Weekly Average*

M T W T F S S

Symptom.......................... Weekly Average*

M T W T F S S

Remember to add Monday to Sunday rating onto your graph on the monthly review page

And add the weekly average to your 3 month graph at the start of this book.

Meds I took this week:

Achievements

Challenges faced

Things to order (medication/equipment/etc)

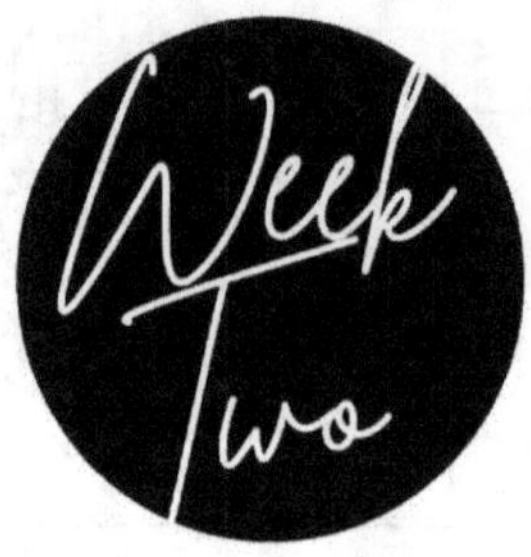

These are your pages to be filled in after a week.

You'll find a medication sheet, timetable, food diary, mood tracker, sleep tracker and dream diary.

These sheets combined keep you organised and in control.

Use these sheets for creating patterns between different things.

Tip: Fill in daily if you think you may not remember, otherwise fill this in on a Sunday eve to be ready for the next week.

PILL / SUPPLEMENT TRACKER

key:

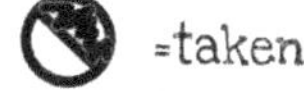
=taken

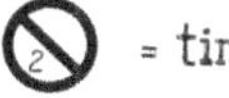
= time

Use different colours for different medications

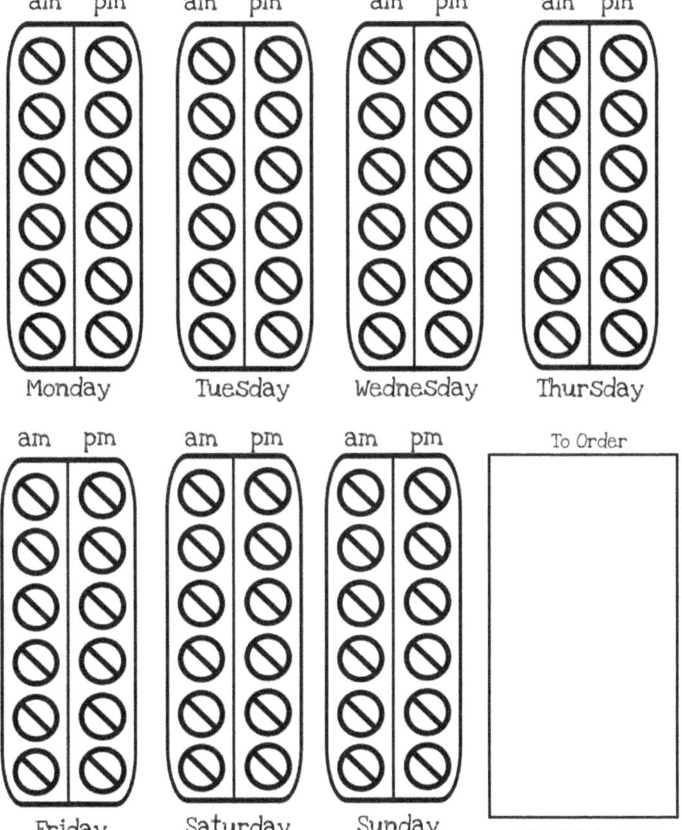

"I can handle anything"

TREATMENT DIARY

Treatment ______________________ Start date: ___________

Date	Dose	pre/post meds taken	Reactions/ side effects	My treat will be

"What doesn't challenge us, doesn't change us"
You can do this.

TREATMENT DIARY

Treatment ____________________ Start date: __________

Date	Dose	pre/post meds taken	Reactions/ side effects	My treat will be

"What doesn't challenge us, doesn't change us"
You can do this.

FOOD DIARY

	Monday	Tuesday	Wednesday	Thursday	Friday	Saturday	Sunday
Breakfast							
Snacks							
Lunch							
Snacks							
Dinner							
Snacks							

HYDRATION TRACKER

Grab a big bottle of water and add the amount of water you've drank in a day.

M	T	W	T	F	S	S

DAILY CHECK IN

Date:..

DAILY 'I AM'S'

Keep them positive! E.g. 'I am able to do anything'

I AM...

I AM...

I AM...

I AM...

I AM...

GRATEFULNESS

Today I am grateful for...

TODAY'S PRIORITIES:

★

★

★

JOURNAL SPACE: What is on your mind today?

SYMPTOMS I FEEL TODAY

Rate each symptom in severity from 1-10. 1 being low and 10 is high

Add these numbers to your monthly review graph

P.S. You can do this!

DAILY CHECK IN

Date:..

DAILY 'I AM'S'

Keep them positive! E.g. 'I am able to do anything'

I AM...

I AM...

I AM...

I AM...

I AM...

GRATEFULNESS

Today I am grateful for...

TODAY'S PRIORITIES:

★

★

★

JOURNAL SPACE: What is on your mind today?

SYMPTOMS I FEEL TODAY

Rate each symptom in severity from 1-10. 1 being low and 10 is high

Add these numbers to your monthly review graph

P.S. You can do this!

DAILY CHECK IN

Date:.......................................

DAILY 'I AM'S'

Keep them positive! E.g. 'I am able to do anything'

I AM...

I AM...

I AM...

I AM...

I AM...

GRATEFULNESS

Today I am grateful for...

TODAY'S PRIORITIES:

★

★

★

JOURNAL SPACE: What is on your mind today?

SYMPTOMS I FEEL TODAY

Rate each symptom in severity from 1-10. 1 being low and 10 is high

Add these numbers to your monthly review graph

P.S. You can do this!

DAILY CHECK IN

Date:..

DAILY 'I AM'S'

Keep them positive! E.g. 'I am able to do anything'

I AM...

I AM...

I AM...

I AM...

I AM...

GRATEFULNESS

Today I am grateful for...

TODAY'S PRIORITIES:

★

★

★

JOURNAL SPACE: What is on your mind today?

SYMPTOMS I FEEL TODAY

Rate each symptom in severity from 1-10. 1 being low and 10 is high

Add these numbers to your monthly review graph

P.S. You can do this!

DAILY CHECK IN

Date:...

DAILY 'I AM'S'

Keep them positive! E.g. 'I am able to do anything'

I AM...

I AM...

I AM...

I AM...

I AM...

GRATEFULNESS

Today I am grateful for...

TODAY'S PRIORITIES:

★

★

★

JOURNAL SPACE: What is on your mind today?

SYMPTOMS I FEEL TODAY

Rate each symptom in severity from 1-10. 1 being low and 10 is high

Add these numbers to your monthly review graph

P.S. You can do this!

DAILY CHECK IN

Date:..

DAILY 'I AM'S'

Keep them positive! E.g. 'I am able to do anything'

I AM...

I AM...

I AM...

I AM...

I AM...

GRATEFULNESS

Today I am grateful for...

TODAY'S PRIORITIES:

★

★

★

JOURNAL SPACE: What is on your mind today?

SYMPTOMS I FEEL TODAY

Rate each symptom in severity from 1-10. 1 being low and 10 is high

Add these numbers to your monthly review graph

P.S. You can do this!

DAILY CHECK IN

Date:...

DAILY 'I AM'S'

Keep them positive! E.g. 'I am able to do anything'

I AM...

I AM...

I AM...

I AM...

I AM...

GRATEFULNESS

Today I am grateful for...

TODAY'S PRIORITIES:

★

★

★

JOURNAL SPACE: What is on your mind today?

SYMPTOMS I FEEL TODAY

Rate each symptom in severity from 1-10. 1 being low and 10 is high

Add these numbers to your monthly review graph

P.S. You can do this!

END OF WEEK REVIEW

Symptom......................................

M	T	W	T	F	S	S	Weekly Average*

Symptom......................................

M	T	W	T	F	S	S	Weekly Average*

Symptom......................................

M	T	W	T	F	S	S	Weekly Average*

Symptom......................................

M	T	W	T	F	S	S	Weekly Average*

Symptom......................................

M	T	W	T	F	S	S	Weekly Average*

Remember to add Monday to Sunday rating onto your graph on the monthly review page

And add the weekly average to your 3 month graph at the start of this book.

Meds I took this week:

Achievements

Challenges faced

Things to order (medication/equipment/etc)

Great news!

You're flying through this book and you're nearly at the end!

Now is a great time to order your next book so you get a seamless transition without a break in your tracking.

Strike now before brain fog strikes!

Go to Amazon and search 'ENabled Warrior Tracker Book'.

By the time your next book arrives, you'll be ready to get straight in. Yay!

You've come so far in the last few months, keep that momentum going, you're doing so well.

You're awesome.

#StayENabled

Jessie Ace x

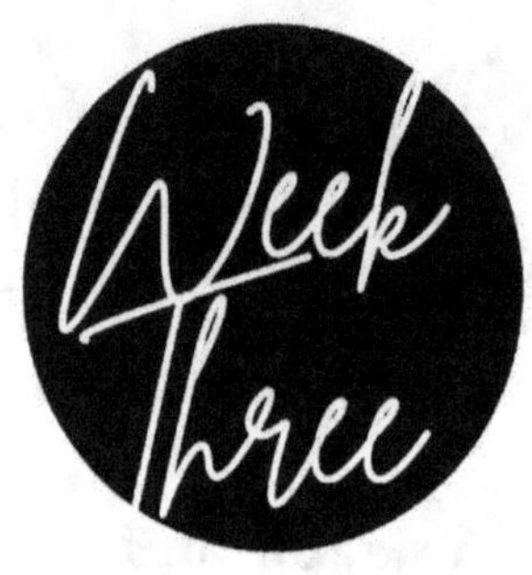

Let's get stuck in to week 3 warrior!

Check through the whole weeks sheets before starting so you don't miss anything

Quote for the week:

How would the person I want to be, do the things that I want to do now?

PILL / SUPPLEMENT TRACKER

key:

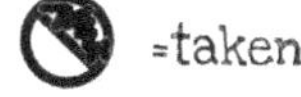

 = time

Use different colours for different medications

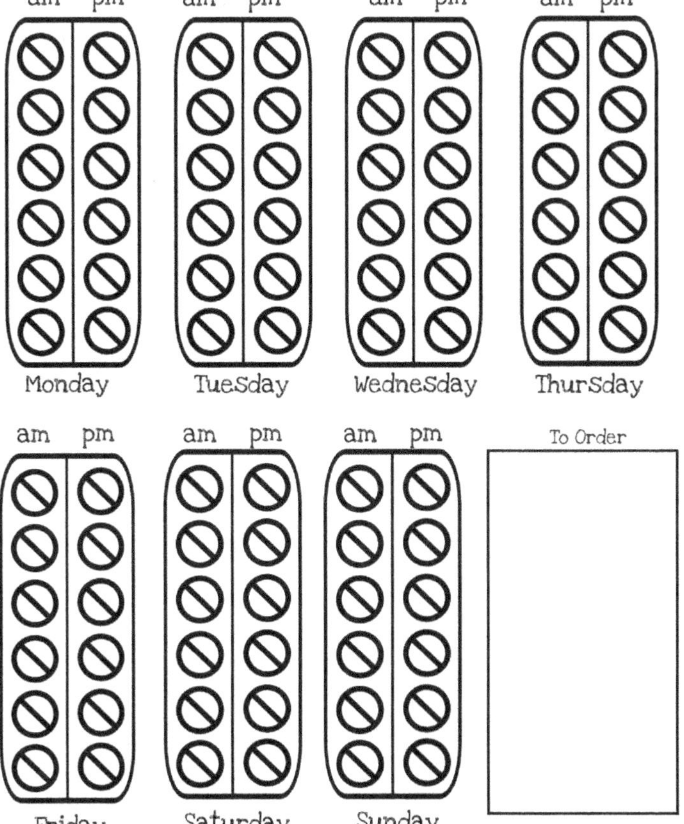

"I can handle anything"

TREATMENT DIARY

Treatment ____________________ Start date: __________

Date	Dose	pre/post meds taken	Reactions/ side effects	My treat will be

"What doesn't challenge us, doesn't change us"
You can do this.

TREATMENT DIARY

Treatment ______________________ Start date: ___________

Date	Dose	pre/post meds taken	Reactions/ side effects	My treat will be

"What doesn't challenge us, doesn't change us"
You can do this.

FOOD DIARY

	Monday	Tuesday	Wednesday	Thursday	Friday	Saturday	Sunday
Breakfast							
Snacks							
Lunch							
Snacks							
Dinner							
Snacks							

HYDRATION TRACKER

Grab a big bottle of water and add the amount of water you've drank in a day.

M	T	W	T	F	S	S

DAILY CHECK IN

Date:..

DAILY 'I AM'S'

Keep them positive! E.g. 'I am able to do anything'

I AM...

I AM...

I AM...

I AM...

I AM...

GRATEFULNESS

Today I am grateful for...

TODAY'S PRIORITIES:

★

★

★

JOURNAL SPACE: What is on your mind today?

SYMPTOMS I FEEL TODAY

Rate each symptom in severity from 1-10. 1 being low and 10 is high

Add these numbers to your monthly review graph

P.S. You can do this!

DAILY CHECK IN

Date:..

DAILY 'I AM'S'

Keep them positive! E.g. 'I am able to do anything'

I AM...

I AM...

I AM...

I AM...

I AM...

GRATEFULNESS

Today I am grateful for...

TODAY'S PRIORITIES:

★

★

★

JOURNAL SPACE: What is on your mind today?

SYMPTOMS I FEEL TODAY

Rate each Symptom in severity from 1-10. 1 being low and 10 is high

Add these numbers to your monthly review graph

P.S. You can do this!

DAILY CHECK IN

Date:..

DAILY 'I AM'S'

Keep them positive! E.g. 'I am able to do anything'

I AM...

I AM...

I AM...

I AM...

I AM...

GRATEFULNESS

Today I am grateful for...

TODAY'S PRIORITIES:

★

★

★

JOURNAL SPACE: What is on your mind today?

SYMPTOMS I FEEL TODAY

Rate each symptom in severity from 1-10 1 being low and 10 is high

Add these numbers to your monthly review graph

P.S. You can do this!

DAILY CHECK IN

Date:...

DAILY 'I AM'S'

Keep them positive! E.g. 'I am able to do anything'

I AM...

I AM...

I AM...

I AM...

I AM...

GRATEFULNESS

Today I am grateful for...

TODAY'S PRIORITIES:

★

★

★

JOURNAL SPACE: What is on your mind today?

SYMPTOMS I FEEL TODAY

Rate each symptom in severity from 1-10. 1 being low and 10 is high

Add these numbers to your monthly review graph

P.S. You can do this!

DAILY CHECK IN

Date:..

DAILY 'I AM'S'

Keep them positive! E.g. 'I am able to do anything'

I AM...

I AM...

I AM...

I AM...

I AM...

GRATEFULNESS

Today I am grateful for...

TODAY'S PRIORITIES:

★

★

★

JOURNAL SPACE: What is on your mind today?

SYMPTOMS I FEEL TODAY

Rate each symptom in severity from 1-10 1 being low and 10 is high

Add these numbers to your monthly review graph

P.S. You can do this!

DAILY CHECK IN

Date:..

DAILY 'I AM'S'

Keep them positive! E.g. 'I am able to do anything'

I AM...

I AM...

I AM...

I AM...

I AM...

GRATEFULNESS

Today I am grateful for...

TODAY'S PRIORITIES:

★

★

★

JOURNAL SPACE: What is on your mind today?

SYMPTOMS I FEEL TODAY

Rate each symptom in severity from 1-10. 1 being low and 10 is high

Add these numbers to your monthly review graph

P.S. You can do this!

DAILY CHECK IN

Date:..

DAILY 'I AM'S'

Keep them positive! E.g. 'I am able to do anything'

I AM...

I AM...

I AM...

I AM...

I AM...

GRATEFULNESS

Today I am grateful for...

TODAY'S PRIORITIES:

★

★

★

JOURNAL SPACE: What is on your mind today?

SYMPTOMS I FEEL TODAY

Rate each symptom in severity from 1-10. 1 being low and 10 is high

Add these numbers to your monthly review graph

P.S. You can do this!

END OF WEEK REVIEW

Symptom.......................

M	T	W	T	F	S	S	Weekly Average*

Symptom.......................

M	T	W	T	F	S	S	Weekly Average*

Symptom.......................

M	T	W	T	F	S	S	Weekly Average*

Symptom.......................

M	T	W	T	F	S	S	Weekly Average*

Symptom.......................

M	T	W	T	F	S	S	Weekly Average*

Remember to add Monday to Sunday rating onto your graph on the monthly review page

And add the weekly average to your 3 month graph at the start of this book.

Meds I took this week:

Achievements

Challenges faced

Things to order (medication/equipment/etc.)

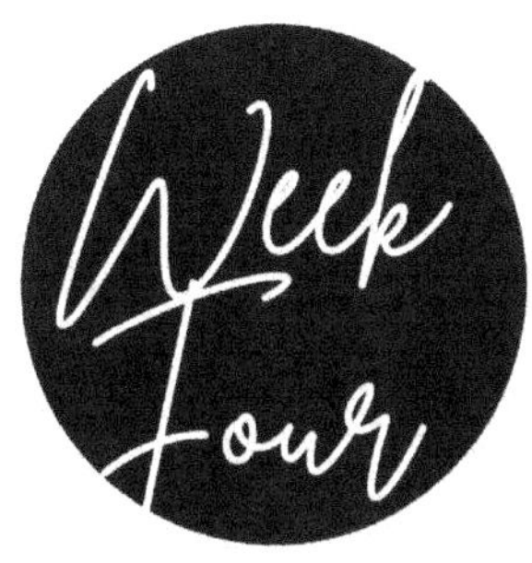

Let's get stuck in to week 4 warrior!

Check through the whole weeks sheets before starting so you don't miss anything

Quote for the week:

As long as you breathe you got a shot at your dream.

PILL / SUPPLEMENT TRACKER

key:

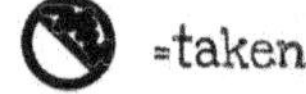
=taken

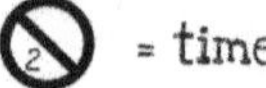
= time

Use different colours for different medications

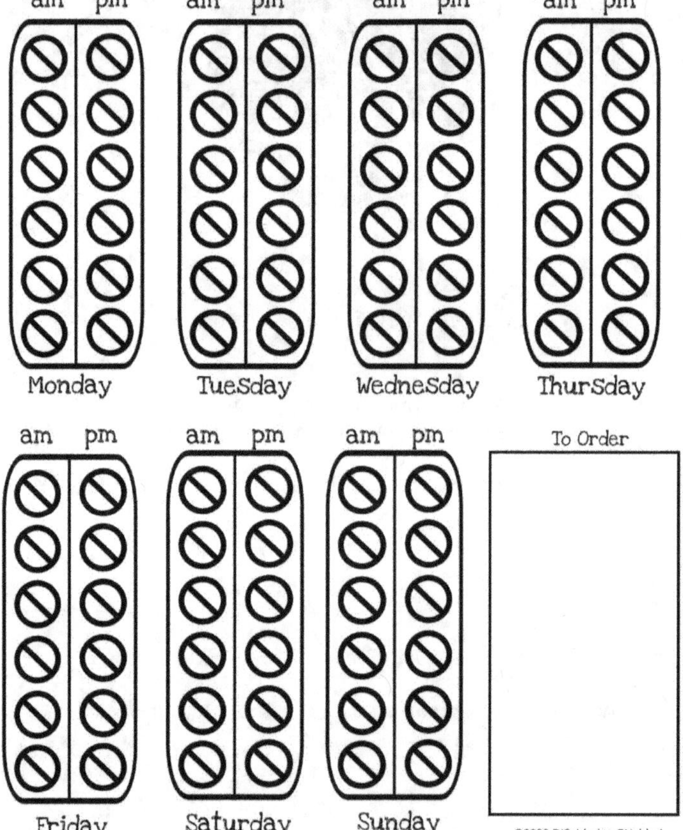

To Order

"I can handle anything"

TREATMENT DIARY

Treatment ______________________ Start date: ___________

Date	Dose	pre/post meds taken	Reactions/ side effects	My treat will be

"What doesn't challenge us, doesn't change us"
You can do this.

TREATMENT DIARY

Treatment ____________________ Start date: __________

Date	Dose	pre/post meds taken	Reactions/ side effects	My treat will be

"What doesn't challenge us, doesn't change us"
You can do this.

FOOD DIARY

	Monday	Tuesday	Wednesday	Thursday	Friday	Saturday	Sunday
Breakfast							
Snacks							
Lunch							
Snacks							
Dinner							
Snacks							

HYDRATION TRACKER

Grab a big bottle of water and add the amount of water you've drank in a day.

M	T	W	T	F	S	S

DAILY CHECK IN Date:..

DAILY 'I AM'S'

Keep them positive! E.g. 'I am able to do anything'

I AM...

I AM...

I AM...

I AM...

I AM...

GRATEFULNESS

Today I am grateful for...

TODAY'S PRIORITIES:

★

★

★

JOURNAL SPACE: What is on your mind today?

SYMPTOMS I FEEL TODAY

Rate each symptom in severity from 1-10. 1 being low and 10 is high

Add these numbers to your monthly review graph

P.S. You can do this!

DAILY CHECK IN

Date:..

DAILY 'I AM'S'

Keep them positive! E.g. 'I am able to do anything'

I AM...

I AM...

I AM...

I AM...

I AM...

GRATEFULNESS

Today I am grateful for...

TODAY'S PRIORITIES:

★

★

★

JOURNAL SPACE: What is on your mind today?

SYMPTOMS I FEEL TODAY

Rate each symptom in severity from 1-10 1 being low and 10 is high

Add these numbers to your monthly review graph

P.S. You can do this!

DAILY CHECK IN

Date:..

DAILY 'I AM'S'

Keep them positive! E.g. 'I am able to do anything'

I AM...

I AM...

I AM...

I AM...

I AM...

GRATEFULNESS

Today I am grateful for...

TODAY'S PRIORITIES:

★

★

★

JOURNAL SPACE: What is on your mind today?

SYMPTOMS I FEEL TODAY

Rate each symptom in severity from 1-10. 1 being low and 10 is high

Add these numbers to your monthly review graph

P.S. You can do this!

DAILY CHECK IN

Date:..

DAILY 'I AM'S'

Keep them positive! E.g. 'I am able to do anything'

I AM...

I AM...

I AM...

I AM...

I AM...

GRATEFULNESS

Today I am grateful for...

TODAY'S PRIORITIES:

★

★

★

JOURNAL SPACE: What is on your mind today?

SYMPTOMS I FEEL TODAY

Rate each symptom in severity from 1-10. 1 being low and 10 is high

Add these numbers to your monthly review graph

P.S. You can do this!

DAILY CHECK IN

Date:...

DAILY 'I AM'S'

Keep them positive! E.g. 'I am able to do anything'

I AM...

I AM...

I AM...

I AM...

I AM...

GRATEFULNESS

Today I am grateful for...

TODAY'S PRIORITIES:

★

★

★

JOURNAL SPACE: What is on your mind today?

SYMPTOMS I FEEL TODAY

Rate each symptom in severity from 1-10. 1 being low and 10 is high

Add these numbers to your monthly review graph

P.S. You can do this!

DAILY CHECK IN

Date:...

DAILY 'I AM'S'

Keep them positive! E.g. 'I am able to do anything'

I AM...

I AM...

I AM...

I AM...

I AM...

GRATEFULNESS

Today I am grateful for...

TODAY'S PRIORITIES:

★

★

★

JOURNAL SPACE: What is on your mind today?

SYMPTOMS I FEEL TODAY

Rate each symptom in severity from 1-10. 1 being low and 10 is high

Add these numbers to your monthly review graph

P.S. You can do this!

DAILY CHECK IN

Date:..

DAILY 'I AM'S'

Keep them positive! E.g. 'I am able to do anything'

I AM...

I AM...

I AM...

I AM...

I AM...

GRATEFULNESS

Today I am grateful for...

TODAY'S PRIORITIES:

★

★

★

JOURNAL SPACE: What is on your mind today?

SYMPTOMS I FEEL TODAY

Rate each Symptom in Severity from 1-10. 1 being low and 10 is high

Add these numbers to your monthly review graph

P.S. You can do this!

END OF WEEK REVIEW

Symptom........................

M	T	W	T	F	S	S	Weekly Average*

Symptom........................

M	T	W	T	F	S	S	Weekly Average*

Symptom........................

M	T	W	T	F	S	S	Weekly Average*

Symptom........................

M	T	W	T	F	S	S	Weekly Average*

Symptom........................

M	T	W	T	F	S	S	Weekly Average*

Remember to add Monday to Sunday rating onto your graph on the monthly review page

And add the weekly average to your 3 month graph at the start of this book

Meds I took this week:

Achievements

Challenges faced

Things to order (medication/equipment/etc)

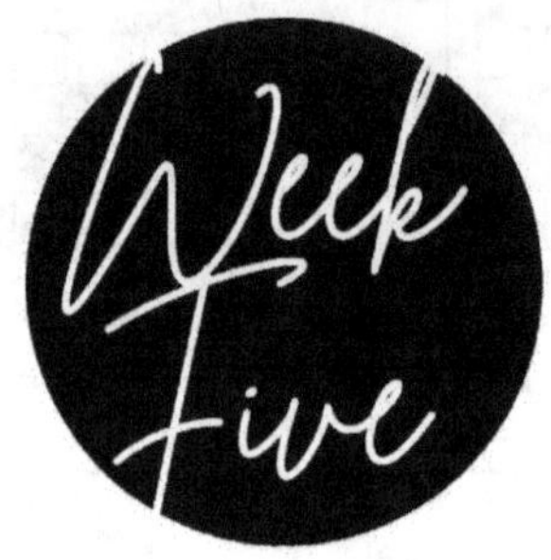

Let's get stuck in to week 5 warrior!

Check through the whole weeks sheets before starting so you don't miss anything

Quote for the week:

Things in life will make you bitter or make you better. You choose which one is the outcome

PILL / SUPPLEMENT TRACKER

key:

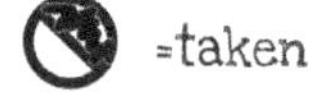

= time

Use different colours for different medications

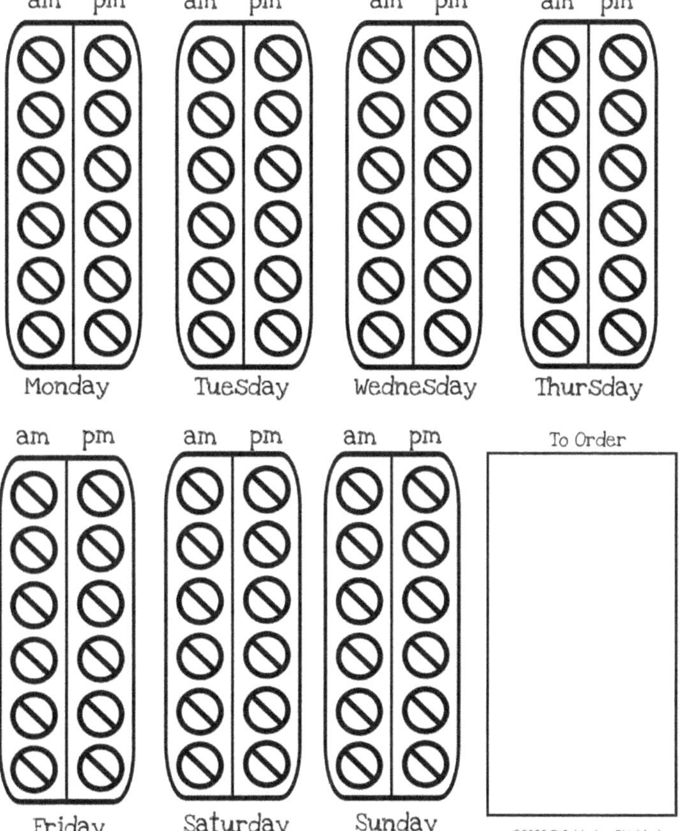

To Order

"I can handle anything"

TREATMENT DIARY

Treatment ____________________ Start date: __________

Date	Dose	pre/post meds taken	Reactions/ side effects	My treat will be

"What doesn't challenge us, doesn't change us"
You can do this.

TREATMENT DIARY

Treatment ______________________ Start date: ___________

Date	Dose	pre/post meds taken	Reactions/ side effects	My treat will be

"What doesn't challenge us, doesn't change us"
You can do this.

FOOD DIARY

	Monday	Tuesday	Wednesday	Thursday	Friday	Saturday	Sunday
Breakfast							
Snacks							
Lunch							
Snacks							
Dinner							
Snacks							

HYDRATION TRACKER

Grab a big bottle of water and add the amount of water you've drank in a day.

M	T	W	T	F	S	S

DAILY CHECK IN

Date:..

DAILY 'I AM'S'

Keep them positive! E.g. 'I am able to do anything'

I AM...

I AM...

I AM...

I AM...

I AM...

GRATEFULNESS

Today I am grateful for...

TODAY'S PRIORITIES:

★

★

★

JOURNAL SPACE: What is on your mind today?

SYMPTOMS I FEEL TODAY

Rate each symptom in severity from 1-10. 1 being low and 10 is high

Add these numbers to your monthly review graph

P.S. You can do this!

DAILY CHECK IN

Date:...

DAILY 'I AM'S'

Keep them positive! E.g. 'I am able to do anything'

I AM...

I AM...

I AM...

I AM...

I AM...

GRATEFULNESS

Today I am grateful for...

TODAY'S PRIORITIES:

★

★

★

JOURNAL SPACE: What is on your mind today?

SYMPTOMS I FEEL TODAY

Rate each symptom in severity from 1-10. 1 being low and 10 is high

Add these numbers to your monthly review graph

P.S. You can do this!

DAILY CHECK IN

Date:...

DAILY 'I AM'S'

Keep them positive! E.g. 'I am able to do anything'

I AM...

I AM...

I AM...

I AM...

I AM...

GRATEFULNESS

Today I am grateful for...

TODAY'S PRIORITIES:

★

★

★

JOURNAL SPACE: What is on your mind today?

SYMPTOMS I FEEL TODAY

Rate each symptom in severity from 1-10. 1 being low and 10 is high

Add these numbers to your monthly review graph

P.S. You can do this!

DAILY CHECK IN

Date:..

DAILY 'I AM'S'

Keep them positive! E.g. 'I am able to do anything'

I AM...

I AM...

I AM...

I AM...

I AM...

GRATEFULNESS

Today I am grateful for...

TODAY'S PRIORITIES:

★

★

★

JOURNAL SPACE: What is on your mind today?

SYMPTOMS I FEEL TODAY

Rate each symptom in severity from 1-10. 1 being low and 10 is high

Add these numbers to your monthly review graph

P.S. You can do this!

DAILY CHECK IN

Date:..

DAILY 'I AM'S'

Keep them positive! E.g. 'I am able to do anything'

I AM...

I AM...

I AM...

I AM...

I AM...

GRATEFULNESS

Today I am grateful for...

TODAY'S PRIORITIES:

★

★

★

JOURNAL SPACE: What is on your mind today?

SYMPTOMS I FEEL TODAY

Rate each Symptom in severity from 1-10. 1 being low and 10 is high

Add these numbers to your monthly review graph

P.S. You can do this!

DAILY CHECK IN Date:...

DAILY 'I AM'S'

Keep them positive! E.g. 'I am able to do anything'

I AM...

I AM...

I AM...

I AM...

I AM...

GRATEFULNESS

Today I am grateful for...

TODAY'S PRIORITIES:

★

★

★

JOURNAL SPACE: What is on your mind today?

SYMPTOMS I FEEL TODAY

Rate each symptom in severity from 1-10. 1 being low and 10 is high

Add these numbers to your monthly review graph

P.S. You can do this!

DAILY CHECK IN

Date:..

DAILY 'I AM'S'

Keep them positive! E.g. 'I am able to do anything'

I AM...

I AM...

I AM...

I AM...

I AM...

GRATEFULNESS

Today I am grateful for...

TODAY'S PRIORITIES:

★

★

★

JOURNAL SPACE: what is on your mind today?

SYMPTOMS I FEEL TODAY

Rate each symptom in severity from 1-10 1 being low and 10 is high

Add these numbers to your monthly review graph

P.S. You can do this!

END OF WEEK REVIEW

Symptom........................

M T W T F S S

Weekly Average*

Symptom........................

M T W T F S S

Weekly Average*

Symptom........................

M T W T F S S

Weekly Average*

Symptom........................

M T W T F S S

Weekly Average*

Symptom........................

M T W T F S S

Weekly Average*

Remember to add Monday to Sunday rating onto your graph on the monthly review page

And add the weekly average to your 3 month graph at the start of this book.

Meds I took this week:

Achievements

Challenges faced

Things to order (medication/equipment/etc)

END OF MONTH REVIEW

Achievements

Challenges faced

Things to order (medication/equipment/etc)

Goal for this month was:

Things to focus on next month

Progress

CONGRATULATIONS

You completed your ENabled Warrior Tracker!

This Tracker book is a lifestyle change not a quick fix, You've come so far in the last 3 months, you are unstoppable!

You've already taken massive action by tracking and managing your symptoms of your chronic illness, how does it feel?

By the way, remember to keep this momentum going and get your next book.

Order now on Amazon.

Search ENabled Warrior Symptom Tracker and remember to write a review for your book on Amazon so that others can find the book.

#StayENabled

Jessie Ace x

www.ingramcontent.com/pod-product-compliance
Lightning Source LLC
Chambersburg PA
CBHW071129260726
48661CB00016BA/838

* 9 7 9 8 7 2 2 3 3 8 9 7 6 *